Dream Time with Children

of related interest

Helping Children to Manage Loss
Positive Strategies for Renewal and Growth
Brenda Mallon
ISBN 1 85302 605 0

Listening to Young People in School, Youth Work and Counselling
Nick Luxmoore
ISBN 1 85302 909 2

Letters to Children in Family Therapy
A Narrative Approach
Torben Marner
ISBN 1 85302 894 0

Helping Children to Build Self-Esteem
A Photocopiable Activities Handbook
Deborah Plummer
ISBN 1 85302 927 0

Understanding Children's Drawings
Cathy Malchiodi
ISBN 1 85302 703 0

How and Why Children Hate
A Study of Conscious and Unconscious Sources
Edited by Ved Varma
ISBN 1 85302 116 4
ISBN 1 85302 185 7

Using Interactive Imagework with Children
Walking on the Magic Mountain
Deborah Plummer
ISBN 1 85302 671 9

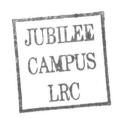
Dream Time with Children

Learning to Dream, Dreaming to Learn

Brenda Mallon

Jessica Kingsley Publishers
London and Philadelphia

First published in the United Kingdom in 2002
by Jessica Kingsley Publishers Ltd
116 Pentonville Road
London N1 9JB, England
and
325 Chestnut Street
Philadelphia, PA 19106, USA

www.jkp.com

Copyright © Jessica Kingsley Publishers 2002

Library of Congress Cataloging in Publication Data
A CIP catalog record for this book is available from the Library of Congress

British Library Cataloguing in Publication Data
A CIP catalogue record for this book is available from the British Library

ISBN 1 84310 014 2

Printed and Bound in Great Britain by
Athenaeum Press, Gateshead, Tyne and Wear

*To my children Karl, Crystal and Danny,
and to all the other wonderful children
who shared their dreams with me.*

Contents

PART ONE

The Basics

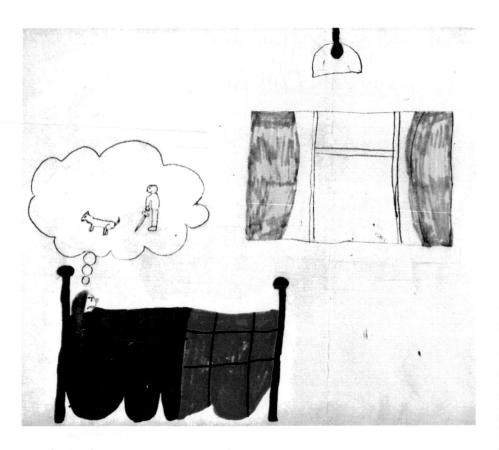

Under Attack

Chapter One

The Eternal World of Children's Dreams

Everyone all over the world dreams. No matter what our culture, our sex, our religion or our race, whether we come from the Sahara Desert or downtown New York, we share the world of dreams. The foetus dreams within the womb, and children spend much of their time in rapid eye movement (REM) or dream sleep. Children need to dream because dreaming is part of the cognitive process where learning is laid down and memories classified and stored. Anyone who cares about their child's progress, emotionally and academically, needs to understand the powerful influence of dreams.

Children are fascinated by dreams. Young children think that dreams come from outside themselves – as one little boy told me, 'they are pictures in my pillow'. He believed that as he slept the pictures rose from his pillow and filled his head with monsters and magic. Later, children become more aware that dreams are part of 'something inside, like when you close your eyes and you see things'. They also become worried about the frightening dreams, the ones in which they feel under attack or alone in strange places. Often children don't talk about these distressing dreams because well-meaning adults say 'Don't worry it's only a dream, it will go away'. Children aren't helped by this dismissal. They may not tell the dream again and may develop problems sleeping, since to sleep means to enter the world of recurring nightmares. If we care for children, we must also care about their dreams.

Why do we dream?

'We dream to rewind our memory.'

Mark (7)

Children are so wise about their dreams. They know that dreams are vital for our well-being, and also that they have a number of essential functions. These were explained by the children and adolescents who took part in research for my book *Children Dreaming*. Later, a film of the same name, which I made for BBC television was shown at the Association for the Study of Dreams conference in 2000. Though the language they used was not particularly sophisticated – they didn't use scientific terms – their essential grasp of the significance of dreaming could not be faulted. In this chapter, I use their explanations to lead us along the path of understanding. Maybe you will recognise your child, or yourself, here.

Dreams help restore our brains

'I think we go into the land of dreams because our brain switches off…it has a rest…it relaxes.'

Camille (7)

Our brains cannot rest while we are awake because then we are in a state of 'quiet readiness', prepared to act if need be. Only when the brain is 'off-line', that is when we sleep, can it rest and be restored; the wear and tear of waking life needs to be repaired in sleep. Sleep and dreaming have played a vital role in our survival: while slow-wave sleep, that is when we are not dreaming, helps repair the body, mental processes like memory consolidation take place during REM sleep. The dream state is a means of recuperation where the neural systems involved in learning, memory, attention and emotional activities are renewed.

At Edinburgh University, Professor Ian Oswald, when researching the effects of drugs such as barbiturates on sleep, discovered that many drugs suppressed dream sleep and once the drugs were no longer administered there was a rebound period of intense, compensatory dream sleep. This lasted about eight weeks, which is the approximate time needed to repair brain cells. He concluded that through dream sleep the brain renews itself. Some drugs prevent this renewal taking place and so the brain valiantly tries to make up the deficit by dreaming avidly once the drugs are stopped. This work is described in *Landscapes of the Night* by Christopher Evans. You may find that your child or the children you work with talk about episodes of 'excessive dreaming'. If so, consider whether medication may be linked in some way.

The REM state makes up the greater part of sleep in newborn babies and children when learning and personality formation is at its greatest. In fact, according to American psychiatrists Ramon Greenberg and Chester Pearlman, premature babies spend as much as 80 per cent of their total sleep time in REM sleep. This decreases with age when, says American sleep researcher Ernest Rossi, the capacity for new learning and personality growth is reduced.

Dreams sort out the events of our day

'If you've read a horrible book or seen something horrible on the TV, you dream about it and that gets it out of your system. Your dream gets rid of it.'

Nathan (11)

Like Nathan, Roxanne (14) recognised this important aspect of dreaming. She said:

'I am sure dreaming is a way of getting rid of all the loose ends of thoughts in our minds. I usually find that I can connect my dreams with something that has recently happened or with something I have seen or heard.'

The scientific reasoning behind the views of Nathan and Roxanne is to be found in the 'computer theory' of dreams. Psychologist Dr Christopher Evans described it in his book *Landscapes of the Night*. In dreaming, he argues, the brain – the human computer – goes off-line and analyses, sorts, classifies and interprets the mass of information and stimuli which flood through our senses every minute of the day. Out-of-date information is updated, while irrelevant data is reclassified. All this cannot be done while we are awake because of the constant influx of information which we have to deal with there and then. People who meditate or deliberately remove themselves from distractions can do some of this work while they are still 'on-line', but most of us do not allow time for that, so it is up to our dreams to do it for us.

> 'Probably your memory has been using things up during the day and after the day's over, it's calming down from all the work and sorting out all the things and putting them in order, a bit like a computer. Dreams are a little movie you can actually see.'
>
> Connor (12)

A central function of dream sleep is vital for processing of data to take place and while we dream the brain attempts to interpret data. Chemical changes also affect REM sleep. Some chemicals are found at decreased levels in certain types of mental conditions such as Down's syndrome, so a Down's syndrome child's REM has unique characteristics.

As evidence to support his theory, Dr Evans points out that newborn babies spend up to 16 out of 24 hours asleep, half of which is paradoxical or dream sleep, while adults spend only 20 per cent of eight hours' sleep in dream sleep. Such long periods are needed so that babies' brains can come to terms with the vast array of stimuli coming from their brand new world.

> 'I think we might dream if we are scared of something and don't tell anyone. They come from the mind.'
>
> Maria (11)

For a great number of children television and videos provide a major source of disturbing 'entertainment' during the day, and dreaming certainly is involved in the processing of the material seen. We will return to this theme in Chapter 6. The research of Greenberg and Pearlman shows that REM sleep plays an important role in assimilating information. They showed, for instance, that opportunity for REM sleep between first and second showings of an emotionally disturbing film reduces emotional disturbance when the film is seen for a second time – dreams allowed the disturbing experience to be processed.

Dreaming helps us to learn

> 'When we learn something our dreams help us to remember it.'
>
> Zara (15)

In some children the learning mechanisms have become damaged or delayed so their dream sleep has a different pattern than that of children without such damage. When we sleep, our brain will pick up noises around us and include them in the dream content; for example, if it is raining on our bedroom window we might dream of a waterfall. However, autistic children do not handle incoming auditory signals in the normal way during REM sleep. Rather, they handle it in the way a newborn baby might, indicating developmental delay, and so their dreams are different. Dr Ernest Hartmann, an eminent American sleep researcher, explains this in *The Functions of Sleep*: 'Those who do not have the neuronal equipment for new learning or acquisition of information show unusually low D [Dream] time whereas those with a capacity for learning or change show high D time' (p.280).

> 'Dreaming helps us get far-back thoughts which are remote and distant in our minds.'
>
> Rosemary (13)

Rosemary has recognised that through dreams we can get in touch with memories and experiences that are forgotten during our waking life.

REM sleep is necessary for the long-term organisation of memory. If we are deprived of dream sleep data-processing cannot take place and it is much harder for us to recall distant events, or even those of the previous day. Without dream sleep we find it hard to concentrate, our memory is poor, we're irritable and, if deprived long enough, we start to behave in a very bizarre manner: the system breaks down. Dreams are the essential interface between the outer world and the inner reaches of the mind.

Dreams help us solve problems

> 'Dreaming is just like thinking in the day except no one disturbs us and we can see things more clearly because we have nothing else to think about.'
>
> Mari (11)

This is a view that Steven Ablon and John Mach endorse in *Children's Dreams Reconsidered*. As psychoanalysts concerned with the manifest, surface content of dreams and the latent or concealed material held within the dream, they believe dreams reflect our attempts to cope with the emotionally important material of that day or from the days just preceding the dream.

The old saying 'sleep on it' implies that while we sleep, problems are worked through and resolved. Children work through emotional difficulties and, particularly as they get older, find that dreams can actually help with practical, perhaps school-related problems. They awake to find they do know the answer to that maths problem after all. The dreaming brain continues to work with all the information it has available.

Dreams are a way of communicating

> 'Dreams tell us what we are really like on the inside. Our subconscious is letting us know what we think.'
>
> Lucy (11)

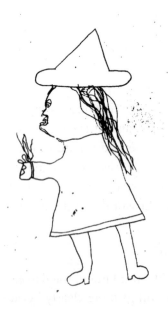

Witch with Hat

Dreams act as an internal information system – they are messages from ourselves to ourselves. They reveal inner struggles and expose the complexity of working out who you are in a confusing world. This is particularly the case for growing children who find that both the physical and emotional changes they experience influence their dream life. This can be seen in 11-year-old Megan's dream: she dreams she is a wolf, but:

> '…a witch puts me under her power and gives me to a werewolf or sometimes the prince of darkness and we go out hunting at night. By day I am a big shaggy dog so no one knows who is killing the people or animals.'

I am sure that few people know that Megan is trying to sort out her confusing desires, her dark (night) and light (day) sides, though her dream communicates these inner conflicts. Another of her dreams makes this even more obvious. She is at that critical time of puberty when she changes physically and emotionally:

> 'The happiest dream I had was when I dreamt that some boys I know called James and Liam were trying to get me down on the ground while we were playing. I turned into a rabbit and ran away, then I turned into a horse. They laughed and jumped on my back. I turned back into a little girl and they went flying into someone's back yard.'

Note how she alters. She changes from scampering rabbit to powerful horse, from being 'sat upon' to 'throwing off' her playful attackers. It is a richly symbolic dream and can be interpreted on a number of levels. Dreams are used in various forms of therapy with children precisely because they communicate unconscious conflicts, anxieties and fears.

Dreams also process waking communications that may have been distressing. One day ten-year-old Carrie's mother told her that she and Carrie's father were going to split up. She told me: 'I dreamt nothing about it for ages then, all of a sudden, I kept having all these really horrible dreams.' She added: 'I wasn't worried about my mum and dad splitting up but I was worried about the dreams.' Those frightening dreams have stopped now because she said: 'We're living in a house on our own now so it's really quite peaceful.'

C.G. Jung, the famous Swiss psychotherapist, believed that dreaming allows us to communicate not only with ourselves and others, but also with the 'collective unconscious', the store of family and racial memories within our psyche. He demonstrated that not only do we dream of things which are personally important and tied in with our own experiences, we also dream of images and symbols which are consciously completely unknown to us. Suddenly, out of the blue, we are hit by a 'big' dream that grips us. We feel it is really significant yet we do not know where it came from or why. There is a flavour of this in 11-year-old Ciara's dream:

> 'The happiest dream I had was when I was walking down the garden of Eden in a pure white flowing dress and I found a baby wrapped in white linen.'

Ciara finds herself in a place of purity, symbolised by the white dress and linen for the child and she is in Paradise. Also, she finds a baby which, in terms of Jungian archetypes, is known as the 'Divine child'. This image figures in dreams across continents, in all age groups and represents human potential and spirituality. There is this heavenly aspect in 10-year-old Sean's dream too:

> 'I flew away to a desert island with my two sisters. The king of the sea came up and lifted the island and he brought us to heaven. There were angels flying about the gate of heaven and I saw the angels welcoming me in.'

Dreams prepare us for the future

> 'When you want to do something you have to dream it first so you know how to do it.'
>
> Alvin (7)

This idea of dreams as a preparation for future action, a rehearsal, is not unusual. Mark (6) dreamt he was going to stay at his friend's house a couple of days before he did so. In the dream he took his pyjama-bag to school and was picked up at the end of the day by his friend's mother. He liked the dream because he felt more confident when facing that first night away from home. The dream acted to prepare and reassure him.

If REM sleep is interfered with, by drugs or sleep deprivation for instance, then we are less able to deal with situations for which we are unprepared. We learn from everything that happens to us during our waking lives, and through dreaming we process and store the information just in case we need it at some future point. We do not 'know' exactly what will happen to us in the future, but nature has found a brilliant way of preparing us for the unexpected.

Dreams let wishes come true

> 'I think we dream because it adds another world to our own and we need another place to escape to. Things can happen in dreams which might never happen in life but you have the experience from the dreams.'
>
> Gwen (15)

Dreaming adds another world to the child's waking world into which she can escape, or which allows her to experience something that is unfulfilled during the day. Erin (8), who lived in a war zone, often has happy dreams. Some of them include her grandmother whom she does not see very often so, at least in the dream, her wish comes true. Similarly, Alex (9), a competition runner, dreamt that he won a race whereas in waking life, there was one boy who always beat him. As he told me gleefully, 'Well, for once I got what I really wanted.'

Escapist dreams of travel, romance, fairyland and favoured TV and pop stars delight children. In them they experience what is not available to them in waking life. Wish-fulfilment dreams are very common and feature in the final chapter, 'Dreamers' Delights'.

> 'I went to a concert to see Kylie Minogue. Then we met outside after it finished. And we were friends.'
>
> Candice (9)

Dreams tell us what is happening when we sleep

> 'I think that while we are asleep we're still thinking and the thoughts become animated instead of just heard. Because we are asleep we're not actually controlling our thoughts, so they

become jumbled up so the characters and places change and dreams don't usually make sense. If you're thinking about something or excited, then you dream that because you're thinking about it so much. Also, if something has happened in the room while you're asleep you dream that. For instance, I was dreaming that I was carrying really heavy weights and when I woke, the cat was sitting on my back and she was heavy.'

Helen (13)

Dreams can be triggered by physical events, like the rain described earlier, but occasionally, like Brett, you can refuse to heed a message! Brett (16) recalled that he frequently wet the bed when younger but he would dream that he was actually in the loo so it was 'all right to wee'. His view was that dreams allow you to get away with things you cannot get away with when awake. The physical pressure of his bladder was communicating to Brett that he needed to urinate. He incorporated this into his dream instead of waking up and going to the toilet.

In a sense, you could see his dream as a way of protecting his sleep: it prevented him from waking up. Freud regarded this protection of sleep as an important function of dreams. As a parent you might find it helpful to explain this idea to your child – if she knows there are explanations for bed-wetting, she may become more relaxed and less anxious. That will help her feelings of self-esteem and, who knows, it might even reduce the bed-wetting!

'One night it was lightning ever so much. My dad left the windows open because it was so hot that night, before the thundering and lightning. Then my mum came in and she closed the windows. I dreamt that my mum was playing the thunder, making the noise, making it happen.'

Jack (12)

These outside influences, outside activities, may come into the dream as Jack described.

Sometimes the impact of the dream causes a physical reaction for the dreamer:

'In my dream I committed a crime and I was hung for it.
When my head came off I fell out of bed.'

Annabelle (10)

Dreams entertain us

We dream because we have nothing to do in bed and are bored.'

Simon (10)

Brian (13) told me: 'We dream so that we don't get fed up while we're asleep.' For him dreaming is a sort of in-house entertainment system! It helps him relax. Like many children, he was quite adamant that we dream in order to prevent boredom.

'We dream because if we have a problem then our dreams try to cheer us up.'

Erin (11)

And finally, one question children may ask is 'Why do I sometimes seem to fall as I am going to sleep?' This is what is known as a 'myclonic jerk'. As the brain is moving over to sleep mode, where major muscles are shut down so we don't kick out in our dreams, it sometimes happens that the process is not as smooth as it should be. It is like changing gear in a car, we may crunch them and this gives us a shudder. Often the child has a sensation of falling or suddenly stumbling. Charles (8) gives us a good example:

'I was a mouse and fell down a grid and then I woke up.'

Children's dream themes

Now we know why children dream, it is time to explore universal dream themes. There is great consistency, historically and culturally, in the subjects children dream about.

'I saw myself walking along a long, dark corridor and suddenly my teacher Mr Jones was creeping up behind me. When I turned round he started throwing maths tests at me, then I woke up.'

Robin (10)

Threatening dream characters are regular, if unwelcome, visitors in dreams. Over time these change from monsters and ghosts to anonymous males and impersonal enemies or, worse, known members of the family. Charles Kimmins, a London inspector of schools, collected a vast number of dream narratives from children in 1918 and it is interesting to compare these with the subjects children dream about today. Are they so different from 1918? He discovered that 25 per cent of the frightening dreams of children under eight consisted 'chiefly of the dread of objectionable men'. Otherwise, apart from dreams of air raids, children today dream of the same subjects. Of course, there were no television or video-influenced dreams then, but books certainly triggered dream imagery.

> 'My most frightening dream ever was when I dreamt that someone was watching me and following me.'
>
> Clodagh (10)

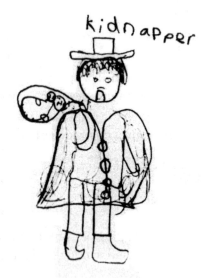

Kidnapper

Typical dream themes found by Kimmins are:

- wish-fulfilment and fear
- kinaesthetic movement (such as floating and flying)

- references to fairy-stories
- bravery and adventure
- school activities
- cinema-influenced
- exciting books
- conversations
- separation.

We will develop 'dream time themes' in Part 2, but first a brief overview of what you are likely to encounter as you spend 'dream time' with children.

Anxiety dreams

> 'We dream because we are worried or nervous about something.'
>
> Jill (10)

Monsters often lurk in children's dreams. Free from the protection and control of the adult's waking world all manner of fears and worries prowl through children's dreamscapes. Dracula, werewolves, Freddy from *Nightmare on Elm Street* and evil kidnappers chase and torment the dreamer. As you can see from the illustrations, these are not beings we would choose to meet if we had the choice.

Conflicts produce anxiety, and dreams both reveal the anxiety and often offer ways to reduce it. This adaptive function of dreams enables the child both to discharge intense emotions and move beyond them.

Being chased or under attack

> 'I dream I get beaten up by people.'
>
> Nigel (10)

In their dreams children find themselves chased through city streets and empty deserts. Sometimes the threat is an animal, such as a lion or wolf, at other times the dreamer is pursued by ghosts, monsters or alien beings. Threats, real and imagined, may be translated into dreams in which the child is hurt or hurts herself. Rosanna's (6) dream was inspired by her fear of pigeons:

> 'I dreamt I was in my house then I went outside and there were lots of pigeons and I was trapped and they kept on biting me. I was trying to get to my mum and when I got to the gate a pigeon was hiding from me and it pecked me.'

These express the vulnerability children do not articulate when awake. In their dreams the imagery reveals fear of being hurt, being powerless and unable to find a protective guardian. Some dreams include elements of chase and attack as Rupert (9) found:

> 'I was lying in bed when it suddenly disappeared. I found myself in a sea with a great white shark swimming towards me. This dream happened again and again and I woke up in a cold sweat.'

In other dreams Rupert himself turns into a shark. He says he has a phobia about sharks.

Some children escape from pursuers by flying away:

> 'A gang of Red Indians were chasing me so I jumped off the canyon and flew down to the ground.'
>
> Nicholas (10)

They escape the pull of gravity, or grave situations, and rise above the danger. This is a very positive response and affirms a sense of personal power and belief in self.

Compensation dreams

> 'We dream to try to make our dreams come true.'
>
> David (10)

Where waking life is lacking, or is perceived by the child as such, then compensation dreams come. David dreams of food because, as he told me, he really likes food but often doesn't feel quite full enough. The dream provides what the child wants in waking life. You sometimes find this with a child whose parents have divorced. 'I dreamt the clock went backwards to the time before my mum and dad separated,' a boy told me. In his dreams he could return to a happier time in his life.

Myths and media

'We dream because we watch television with a nightmare on.'

Jane (10)

There are supposedly only seven stories in the world and all the books, films, TV serials and legends are variations on these original themes. In children's dreams we see the influence of these stories, like this one which has elements of the theme of deep sleep and awakening in a changed world, such as we see in *Rip Van Winkle* and *Snow White*.

'I was riding my bike and a dog came after me. Then a kind of green ghostly man jumped out and put me in a deep sleep. He brought me to his cave and threw me in a dog's den. Then I woke up and thought the dog was in my room.'

Stephanie (10)

The cave image recurs for Mattie (10). There is the element of having to go to the symbolic depths in order to find what he most desires:

'I went into a large, dark cave and walked and walked and walked until I came to an archway. Inside the archway was loads and loads of gold which I could keep.'

Children are heavily influenced by television and videos, which expose them to vast amounts of stimuli that pervade their dreaming world.

'When we watch films they make you scared and you dream about the film again.'

Janet (10)

'Films and videos make me dream of killing and war.'

David (10)

Animals

> 'The most frightening dream was of a dog and when he came up
> to me a snake came out of his mouth but every time he tried to bite
> me, I got away.'
>
> Nicholas (10)

Animals are important to children and whilst in dreams they may represent
real animals often they are a disguise for people or feelings. For example,
the dog and the snake may symbolise a person who is frightening
Nicholas, perhaps someone who is being venomous and verbally attacking
him. We will return to animals again and again as we travel the world of
children's dreams.

Problem-solving

> 'I think we dream because when we need to sort out a problem or
> have something on our minds it causes us to have stress and we
> have to think it over and the stress causes us to dream.'
>
> Nicci (10)

Whilst we sleep our brains continue to gnaw away at issues that are of
concern to us. Great scientists have spoken of the power of their dreams
which enabled them to make startling breakthroughs. Friedrich Kekulé
von Stradomitz, who discovered the benzene ring, said as he concluded his
report to the Benzole Convention (1890): 'Gentlemen, let us learn to
dream', quoted in van der Castle 1994, p.36.

But which is the reality – dreaming or waking?

Catherine (13) told me that when she was younger she used to think that
when she was dreaming it was really happening to a little girl in America,
and during the day what happened to Catherine was really that other girl's
dreams! Many adults also have commented on that aspect of dreaming.
Which is the 'real' world: the one we dream of or the one in which we are
awake? The answer is that these two worlds are both essential to life, as
without either one we could no longer be fully alive.

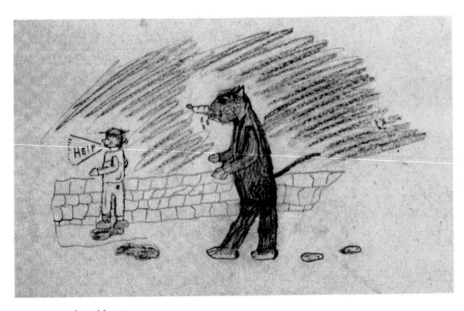

Boy Being Chased by Bear

Chapter Two

Ages and Stages

For the Mae Enga [of New Guinea], the dream is not inside the individual but rather the individual finds himself inside the dream. This concept of the dream is not unlike that which Piaget finds common in young children.

Carl W. O'Neill, *Dreams, Culture and the Individual*

As children develop, so do their dreams. Just as children grow at their own pace, so their dreams parallel the stages of waking cognitive development. In this way, dreaming is a cognitive act, reorganising memories in the dream narrative and its images. In a way children's dreams are illustrated stories which help them to learn about living. The stages outlined below provide a rough guide to what dreams you might meet in your dream time with children. However, dreaming starts long before a toddler first talks of dreams.

Dreaming in the womb

Research into the whole area of dreaming and its significance in early childhood development, reported by British researchers Francis Crick and Graeme Mitchison, concludes that dreaming takes place in the womb, especially in the last trimester, when the foetus matures and develops highly complex processes essential for independent survival. It is as if

REM sleep within the womb lets the baby prepare for or 'anticipate' his future world. REM sleep is also essential because it stimulates the central nervous system, which helps prepare for later structural growth. REM sleep provides a mechanism for the establishment of neural pathways in the brain. Newborn babies need far more REM sleep than adults. As adults we do not need to dream as much as neonates do, because those pathways have already been laid down. Unfortunately we cannot ask babies what they dream about, we can only observe and make our own guesses. But as their language develops, so toddlers can tell us about their dreams.

What do toddlers dream about? Ages 2–3 years

'The earliest dream I remember was about a yellow dragon that could breathe fire out of its tail, nose, mouth and left foot.'

Cathy (8)

Very young children often have difficulties separating dream reality from waking reality. Up to the age of 3 children say that dreams come from God, the television or fairies or that they are 'pictures in my pillow'. This changes gradually, so that by 6 or 7 children begin to accept that dreams happen in their own heads, not 'out there'; they learn to distinguish between the outside world of reality and the inner world of dreams.

Children in this age group may not be able to talk about their dreams, and those with special educational needs or developmental delay may be limited in their ability to describe and relate their dreams. Because language is still fairly restricted at this age, it is not until 3 and 4 that we begin to get a fuller picture of those 'pictures in my pillow'. Even then there are many 2- and 3-year-olds who think that dreaming happens whenever you lie in bed and close your eyes – whether or not you have fallen asleep!

Marigold (4) attends a tiny school in a remote rural area. The farm on which she lives provides a lot of her dream imagery; indeed Marigold told me that her dreams come not from her head but 'from the fields' outside her window. She had a nightmare recently in which a 'biting tiger' was coming out of the cupboard in her bedroom. Like many youngsters she sometimes lies awake imagining that all sorts of dangers inhabit her room, and these fears surface in dreams.

Some 3-year-olds may be describing sophisticated dreams while some others may never mention them at all. Nightmares often appear at 3 years of age and continue to be highly represented right through to 16; however, in this book I'll concentrate on dreams of children up to the age of 13.

Pre-school dreams: Ages 4–5 years

In the pre-school years all sorts of conflicts arise, particularly as the child has to learn to control their instinctive, ego-centred side and learn to live within the norms of their social group. This is a demanding time, and dreams reveal the inner conflict of this transition – the socialisation process can be very difficult for adults and children alike.

Lucinda (12) recalled dreams of conflict she had when she was 4 years old!

> 'I used to have [dreams about] models from a shop window my mum used to take me to. I was only about 4 at the time when I started having them but I had them every night until I was about 8. There were two models, one with red hair and the other had white hair. The redhead was evil and used to try and lead me into bad ways. The other was quiet but also bad. Different things happened every night. It doesn't sound scary but when you're four it is.'

We can see how temptation here symbolises the inevitable struggle between the different parts of ourselves. We are incredibly complex beings, children and adults alike. We each have a central core but, like a diamond, we are all many-faceted. Dreams allow us to experience aspects of ourselves that we may never have time to consider during the day. Children want to be both good and bad, and dreams reflect this pull.

The projection of feelings on to other characters in the dream drama, as with the red-haired and white-haired mannequins is not done at a conscious level. In television programmes, in films and in books children see and 'recognise' the struggle between the good guy and the evil invader, and they learn how hard a time characters like the three little pigs have against the greedy wolf. All this mirrors their internal struggles to be good and conform while still being sorely tempted to be naughty. The character Pinocchio is a lovely example of this tug of war.

> 'I had a dream about some evil spirits coming in my bedroom and throwing my toys on the floor and breaking some of them and they ripped the curtains down. Then they went downstairs and we could not see anyone. Then I woke up and all my toys were back.'
>
> Heather (8)

When Heather woke up she was surprised that the toys had been put back. Dreams feel just as real as waking events for many children, just as they do for adults.

Young children dream of monsters, ghosts and fairies, indeed the world of fairies is usually associated with childhood. On the one hand fairyland is a land of magic and fantasy, but on the other hand it is the land of nature. Fairies live in forests and dells, in woodlands and by streams. They live in a highly structured society like our own, and there are kings and queens and laws which can be enforced. There are good and bad fairies, just like people, and children identify with fairies in their magical world and dream of them.

Animals are almost always present in the dreams of children. The cats, dogs, wolves and birds that feature in these dreams very often stand in place of the dreamer. It is much 'safer' to project all our angry feelings on to a mad dream-bull for instance, than to acknowledge just how destructive we feel. However, in the case of 6-year-old Ivan Mishukov his dreams reveal a much closer connection. He was abandoned by his mother and adopted by a pack of dogs outside Moscow. He was with them for two years and now they and dreams of them obsess him constantly, as reported in *The Observer* in 1998. 'I was better off with the dogs,' he said. 'They loved and protected me.'

Witches too symbolise the conflict between good and bad: traditionally the black-clad witch represents evil. The witch figure is an age-old stereotype devised in response to the fear of the unknown powers of the archetypal, untamed 'wise woman'. In dreams of witches, children express the stereotype found in Grimms' fairy-tales, for example. Witches are also used in dreams to symbolise mothers, especially if the child has just had a row with her mother and is feeling particularly angry. Many of the themes pre-school children dream about are developed as they grow and mature. Let us see how these change.

First steps to independence: Ages 5–7 years

> The dreams of young children are vivid and very real. A boy of six dreamt someone had given him a threepenny piece and on waking he searched the bed for it.
>
> Charles Kimmins

Many of you will know that bittersweet feeling as you see your child go to school for the first time. As you leave her behind it feels as if a new stage of life has begun and tears are shed not just by the child, if she cries at all, but by the parent too. The process of separation is truly under way. In this transitional stage, where the child moves into a more independent world of school and stronger relationships with peers, dreams develop a sequential narrative, a storyline that contains images and kinaesethetic elements – bodily sensations such as flying.

Children at this stage also become more aware that bad, unpredictable events can happen. Someone in the family might, for example, get sick or leave, and their dreams highlight this awareness. Their fear of separation sometimes translates into dreams of being abandoned by their mother.

> 'I had a dream about my mum being in hospital.'
>
> Jyoti (6)

Five-year-olds told me over and over again about their dreams of ghosts and monsters. In the main, other subjects were witches, animals – wild, tame and mythical – immediate family and being hurt in some way.

> 'One night I dreamt a vampire came into my house and bit my mum and me.'
>
> Kerry (6)

At this age there is still occasional difficulty in distinguishing between dreaming and waking reality, but largely children know that they dream, even though they may still believe the dreams come from the outside world.

'I had a dream about a witch and she put a spell on me and turned me into a frog and I went croak.'

Sal (6)

A universal theme that may emerge at this stage is that of being chased. The pursuer may not be a person though. When Sally was 6 she dreamt about a washing machine that chased her around the room, then she dreamt about a malevolent toilet:

'I used to dream about toilets opening and closing and eating people up whenever they used them. I dreamt that they filled up with water when someone shuts the door after they've used it. I dreamt that I'd used it, went out and remembered that I'd left something in there and went back. The door slammed I couldn't get out and I drowned.'

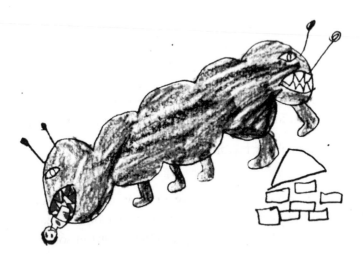

twice a giant caterpillar squashed my house and it is eating me

Caterpillar Eating Me

It is easy to lose sight of the fact that things we take for granted, like toilets and washing machines, can be seen as noisy, frightening presences that seem have a life of their own.

Christopher (6) dreamt of a ferocious giant two-headed caterpillar which squashed his house and then ate him. His dreams affected his waking behaviour as they do for many children. For instance, he dreamt that there was a monster in his mother's bag, and next day he would not go near it, skirting round his mother when out shopping, just to avoid contact. His mother wondered why he was behaving so strangely, until he told her about the dream. The line between dreams and reality is still very thin at this stage of a child's development.

Dreams of bravery and adventure are not found too often in this age group. Keziah (6) was a rare example, for she has a particularly empowering dream. In it, she says:

> 'I can change into anything I want and do anything. I changed into the strongest person in the world and I went to help people in fires.'

Moving on: Ages 7–9 years

There is more of an edited quality about dreams at this stage. Rather than a camera left running as in the earlier stage, here the child has a character who 'sees' the dream and takes part in the dream activity. There are more dreams about people outside the family and strangers who are 'bad' or threatening in some way. Despite their growing independence children still feel vulnerable as their dreams reveal:

> 'The most frightening dream I've had was when I got kidnapped by two men and they drove me away to a forest and kept me there for a week.'
>
> Cassandra (7)

> 'The most frightening dream I have had is about my sister on her tricycle riding on to the road and someone sees her and takes her away and I can't stop thinking about that.'
>
> Umza (9)

Children wrestle with feelings of powerlessness. Claudette (7) is ultimately successful in her dream struggle but it involves enormous effort to be so:

> 'I dream about my sister. It is a terrible dream. Leanne sat on the chair near the window, she's like at the pictures. Someone was near the window. It was a ghost. He strangled her. She was flat dead on the floor, but he was still strangling her. I was near and asleep. I woke up and saw her on the floor. I woke up crying but she was in her bed.'

She described another dream in which her sister again features centrally:

> 'I dreamt about the devil. We all went down to the devil. He wouldn't let us go so he said, dig in the garden. I was sweating, then we found a knife. We sneaked in the house and stabbed the devil and we went back up, we were glad.'

In some families where there is a great deal of upset, brothers and sisters dream of helping each other and of sticking together against the world. Claudette's sister is her lifeline, so her dream tells us of her extreme anxiety about her sister being hurt. In the final dream, together they overcome the life-threatening evil but they have to go down to the depths to do so. In Jungian terms they seek a solution in the dark world of emotion. It would be of little use for Claudette to seek a solution in her head – in the attic as it is often symbolised in dreams – because it is gut instinct for survival and her animal sweat which will get her through.

Such assertive action is unusual at Claudette's age as sleep researcher Louise Ames has explained. Though fear dreams start early, it is usually not until 7 that the child begins to fight back. Also, at this time he starts to become the central active figure, and not just the recipient of the action: he moves from passive to active. Also, fears take on a different dimension, the child begins to fear things especially about himself at about 7 years of age. Whereas earlier he was worried that his mother would be separated from him, at 7 fears and worries are real personal fears about himself. This is not surprising, since 7 is the age when the child is consolidating his own sense of self and naturally he worries about his survival. Nicholas (7) called this his 'true nightmare':

'I dream about another lady that looks like my mum, and she wants to kill me. She tries to trick me that's she's my real mum and one day she tricked me by picking me up from school. And she was walking down Dover Street with me and my real mum came and they started arguing saying I was their son then the lady got out a knife and killed my mum and she turned round and was just about to kill me then I woke up and I never knew who my real mum was.'

Between the ages of 5 and 12 most children experience troublesome nightmares at some time. Nightmares are upsetting for children and parents alike and the child may find that the feelings they provoke may linger for days. Emma (10) gives a fine example of this:

'Once when I was sick I dreamt that my sister was Dracula and for weeks after that I refused to sleep in the room with her. She teased me by showing her teeth.'

Times of change: Ages 10–13 years

Rapidly changing physical characteristics and hormonal changes during this stage can induce many dreams of insecurity. They revolve round health, school, personal harm, family and personal relationships, and they reflect the increased independence the child seeks. Children also worry about war, disasters and the environment.

Though dreams about school are generally not prevalent in early childhood, at this transition stage and at times of examinations however, they become much more apparent. Louise (11) had a terrifying dream about school:

'The dream which is the most terrifying I have ever had is, me and my brother went to this science lesson and we sat down, and when my brother got something wrong, the teacher pulled this lever and he fell down a trap door and fell onto this thick knife, and it went through his stomach.'

Louise is not looking forward to leaving her present small school. She has been the subject of older pupils' mythology-mixed-with-the-truth tales in which the 'new kid' is subjected to horror stories guaranteed to scare.

Louise needs assurance about her new school: talking through these anxieties would help.

Many children in this age group dream of literally being left on their own, as Nasreen (11) does:

> 'I once dreamed about my brother drowning in the shower, because I told him not to play with water, he disobeyed me and died. After that I dreamt about all my family walking to London airport to go to India. I was too slow and lost my way.'

Rosaleen (11), described her most frightening dream:

> 'I dreamt about going home but my brother runs away from me, and when I get home none of my family knows me and I travel around, nowhere to go. So, I go to my friend's house but they think I am a stranger and close the door in my face.'

The price Nasreen and Rosaleen pay for not being able to take on the adult role is the loss of a brother and the desertion of a family. Guilty feelings about inability to care adequately for others are found particularly in the dreams of girls.

Dreams where everyone else has died and the dreamer is the only person left alive are common around puberty. In some cases the family leaves, while in others tragedy strikes, such as all the dreamer's family is killed in a car crash so he is left to fend for himself. Far less frequent are dreams in which the dreamer is overtly aggressive; usually he is the target, but for 12-year-old Denise this is not the case:

> 'My most frightening dream… Well, I woke up crying because I dreamt that I was a murderer and killed all my family.'

She was shocked by the violence, the intensity of her antagonism. Animal-mad Claire (11) dreams, when she is ill, that she will die and 'never see my mum and dad and my pets ever, ever again'. She had another dream in which:

> 'I met some elves and they were bad but I never knew, they looked so innocent. I was lost and they offered me some bread and milk. It was poisoned. They started to run round in a circle saying, "She's dead, she's dead, the little girl is dead".'

Fear of being harmed or permanently damaged is a real fear for many children.

> 'I dreamt I was kidnapped from school and left to die.'
>
> Victoria (10)

> 'I have horrible dreams about snakes crawling up my bed and trying to kill me.'
>
> Helen (13)

Family dynamics

Families can be warm and loving, cruel and destructive, a mixture of all of these or just 'good enough' – good enough to nourish our children so they have an adequate sense of self-worth and confidence to make their way in the world. For most children the family is where we start from, where we begin to have a sense of who we are. The importance of the secure caring unit, be it single-parent or wide, extended family, is crucial. We can see from the following dreams how the child's perception of family dynamics is communicated through dreams:

> '...they turned into baddies and tried to get me. I was frightened. All the family changed into baddies except me.'
>
> Giorgio (5)

Giorgio had the dream after his parents had been cross with him. In the dream he sees their faults, for they are 'the baddies', while he is good. Bob (7), whose parents recently split up, has wish-fulfilment dreams in which an anonymous professor builds a space ship that takes the boy to China where his father is waiting. Absent parents frequently figure in the dreams of children whose parents, or parental figures, have separated.

Chandra (7) who has a baby brother had a nightmare which made her cry:

> 'A baby monster took my baby away to his castle. The monster's mum came and took my baby away and I never saw my baby, ever.'

Many young children call their baby brother or sister 'my baby', as Chandra does. Possessiveness, affection and a sense of responsibility towards the younger sibling mix together, and fears surface in the dreamscape.

Between ages 8 and 10 many children like to talk about dreams, and if wakened in the middle of one try to go back and finish it. They talk to mothers rather than fathers about their dreams, though by about 13, friends are more often chosen as the audience. The dreamer is generally the central actor of the dream, while friends and family continue to play major roles. Wish-fulfilment dreams continue but become more tied to social goals, as Amir's (8) dream shows: Amir dreams he can speak good English and can play football; if he could do these things in his waking life, he believes the other boys at school would accept him.

> 'I dream about fairies having a party. They fly up and down in the air. The queen of fairies is always sitting on her throne and drinking wine all the time!'
>
> Claire (11)

Alicia (8), too, has pleasurable, fairy-tale dreams of princes and kings and queens. Indeed, she was quite unusual in that she could not recall ever having a nightmare. This optimism is to be seen in the reason she gave for dreaming. She said: 'We dream to make people loving and kind.' In other dreams told to me children have found themselves rescued from danger by parents or kind relatives, reflecting their sense of trust in these adults.

Children at this stage may also omit certain parts of the dream which they think are 'stupid' or which may be rejected by adults and get them into trouble. Censorship of dreams is common since all of us really prefer that others think well of us; even St Augustine refused to tell his superiors his dreams because of their 'lewd' nature! So it's important to reassure children that dreams do not have a sense of right and wrong and the dreamer will not be punished for his dreams.

Differences in age and sex

There are differences in dreams according to the child's sex as well as age. David Foulkes's (1977) longitudinal research into this shows no signifi-cant differences in the dreams of pre-school boys and girls; animals and monsters are themes common to both. However, there comes a marked sex-difference in dream content at ages 5 to 6. Then, Foulkes finds boys' dreams are more likely to be centred on conflict, often with male strangers or untamed animals, whereas girls have more friendly dream relationships. As the years pass, similarities and differences continue to emerge in their dreams. These reflect the way in which boys and girls experience and view the world differently.

Between the ages of 8 and 11, girls generally talk about their dreams at greater length because of their superior verbal skills, and their dreams reflect the importance of relationships with family and peers. As American psychologist Sharon Saline wrote in her 1999 paper 'The most recent dreams of children ages 8–11': '...girls are more willing to silence themselves rather than risking relationships due to an argument.'

Sibling rivalry

Sibling rivalry is annoyingly normal though often difficult to live with. However, the arguments competition between siblings does have a positive side. Many psychologists would argue that it helps children to learn interpersonal skills including those of negotiation and survival. Children learn these within the family and then use them in the outside world of school and later, at work.

As with all close relationships, there are times when intense feelings become out of control. They may cause arguments and fights. Dreams often reveal underlying concerns that children have about their brothers and sisters, whether or not they are expressed in waking hours. They also blend past expereices, 'old hurts', with present ongoing experiences to create the dream narrative, In many instances, negative feelings about siblings are thinly disguised, as we see with Gideon's dream:

> 'I dreamt our house was bombed and that we ran away and hid. Then loads of soldiers came into the house looking for us. We discovered we'd left my older brother behind, then I woke up!'
>
> Gideon (10)

On one level he certainly would like to leave his brother behind, but pressure from family and society ensures that he does not voice such a wish too loudly. Similarly Sinead (8) dreams that a bomb killed her elder brother, whom she says she hates, when he went away on an army posting and she was relieved to hear the news. In another of her dreams he turned into a dog. No love lost there!

> 'I dreamt that "Psych" was my brother and when my mum and dad went out he tried to kill me.'
>
> Annie (10)

Some dreams are about a separation devoutly wished for, as is the case for Dawn (12). She lives with her mother and father and two brothers and described her happiest dream as one in which her brothers moved out and she 'had peace' and a room to herself!

Common dream themes

A common anxiety dream for Lisa (12) is that one by one her teeth fall out. Insecurity about looks and separation, 'falling out' with friends and relatives is often the trigger for this type of dream.

Falling dreams are found at all ages and may signify feelings of being out of control or that we need to let go. Some children believe the superstition that if you hit the ground in a falling dream, you will die, so it is important to assure them that this does not happen. Siri (13) dreams that he does not fall himself, but that his clothes do!

> 'I dreamt I got up late and didn't have time to get dressed and so I went out with no clothes on and keep trying to get covers to cover me up, but they keep falling off.'

> 'I had a dream that I was falling off a cliff into a dark, dark hole and there was a load of snakes in the bottom trying to get me.'
>
> Ellie (13)

Many children feel that sex is a taboo subject, as those who wrote to best-selling author Judy Blume explained in *Letters to Judy: What Kids Wish They Could Tell You.* They feel parents are embarrassed when it comes to sex. In the following examples you can see the sexual dimensions of children's dreams:

Six-year-old Leila has no time for any 'lovey-dovey' stuff:

'I dream about some boys kissing me in the playground. I don't like it.'

Michael (11) dreams of ghosts, space and super-heroes, but he also has what he describes as 'rude' dreams:

'The rude dream is about me getting a girlfriend and taking her to a disco and taking her to my place...' [No more details!]

Clare (9):

'I dreamt about Robbie Williams coming up to me and kissing me and taking me out. I went and we had a great time.'

There were many dreams reported by girls which were suffused in a pink romantic glow: whether inspired by books, television or films, the rose-coloured fantasies continue. Renata (13) has a slightly different angle though:

'I dreamt about my honeymoon night. I was a man and I had to sleep in a pink bed with yellow wallpaper. But I didn't get round to doing "it".'

In the next chapter we will explore the way in which we can share 'dream times' with children.

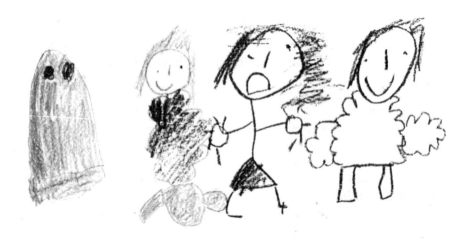

Ghosts and Girls

Chapter Three

Dream Sharing
A Practical Guide

In spite of fear dreams, children...delight in dreaming, and it is an evident pleasure to them to talk about and record their dreams.
Charles Kimmins, *Children's Dreams*

Children enjoy talking about their dreams when they trust the listener or listeners. Surprised as they sometimes are by their own dreamscapes, they often want reassurance from others that they are not weird. Dream sharing provides a chance to reassure, to exchange dreams, to talk through the concerns they raise and to celebrate their exuberant creativity.

One way to encourage the understanding of dreams is to start a dream group. Those who work with children in settings such as residential homes, hospitals and schools where tutorial work takes place will already know of the great insights children gain from sharing with peers, for instance in 'circle time'. Working in a group gives children a place where their dreams can be treated seriously and sensitively, and children of all ages can benefit from dream sharing.

In essence, working with dreams involves:

- communicating
- exploring
- empathising

- imagining
- identifying
- valuing
- sharing.

Starting a dream group

Dreams do not have a moral code, they are uncensored expressions of ideas and feelings, and as such are not subject to our waking codes. We need constantly to bear this in mind so that we do not make judgemental remarks about the dreams that children tell us. Passing negative judgements will make them feel guilty, which in turn makes them clam up, so they refuse to talk about dreams because they are afraid of what you might say. So, bearing that in mind, what do you do if you want to start a group where children can talk about dreams?

Think about the aim of the group

The simple aim may be to provide an opportunity for children to share dreams and to understand themselves more clearly as they understand their dreams. However, if you work with a specialised group, such as children with depression, you may need to consider what other aims you might have. In such a group an objective might be to enable the group members to face their fears or to identify strong 'helpers' in their dreams, or to provide an opportunity for them to explore emotional aspects of their dreams that are repressed or depressed during waking life.

Time spent considering why you are setting up a group and what you hope to achieve is very worthwhile; it makes all the other stages much clearer and easier.

Who will be in the group?

You may decide to have a group where the children are all around the same age, or if it is a family group there may be a spread of ages. What is important to remember is that different things are appropriate and significant to different ages. An adolescent may want to talk about why he has a wet dream, while a 6-year-old may be totally obsessed by monster dreams; and each may be inhibited by the other.

Different levels of verbal ability and understanding are factors you should also consider. By this I do not mean whether they share the same mother tongue, but whether they can share ideas and appreciate what other people in the group might be getting at.

The best group size

If you want to give everyone a chance to work on dreams in any depth, then you need to keep the group small; seven or eight is enough. Having said that, you can work with larger groups, for example a whole class of children, but the work will probably not be in the same depth. In larger groups you, as the group facilitator/enabler, will not have much time to pick up the wide variety of issues that may be raised during any one session.

If you have to work with a large group, give children the opportunity to talk in small groups or in pairs. Also, be aware that children may want to spend time with you if they do not understand their dreams or are troubled by what has been revealed during a dream-group session.

Decide dates and time

Clearly, the time has to be convenient for the group members. Very young children are often tired at night so that is not a good time for them. Choose a time to which everyone can make a regular commitment. Obviously, people get ill and sometimes cannot attend a meeting, but emphasise the importance of regular attendance, otherwise the group finds it hard to bond and some participants feel devalued.

You will need to decide how long the group will run. Will it be open-ended and ongoing, or will it run for, say, ten weekly sessions? Be realistic about the time you can afford. It is useful to have a time limit with children, but there is nothing to stop you renegotiating when the time is up; that way you have a chance to review how the group has gone and to recruit new members if old ones leave.

Two hours is a suitable amount of time for a children's dream group, longer than that is too demanding. For younger ones the sessions may be much shorter and can involve other activities, such as drawing. Be guided by your knowledge of the children involved. Dream-work is work on our emotional selves, and that is very draining, so be sensitive to signs of tiredness.

Choose a venue

The room should be welcoming with comfortable chairs arranged in a circle. It should be private and free of interruptions or onlookers. Also it is useful to have some tables, paper and paints or pencils available for when you do dream drawings.

Define the boundaries

It is important to work out boundaries: first for you, so that you know what issues you feel comfortable with and can cope with; and second for children, because boundaries help children feel secure. So if you are running a group in a school, the children need to know that it is all right to talk about it should they dream of a teacher in an uncomplimentary light! This and the following issues can be dealt with at the first meeting.

Confidentiality

A contract of confidentiality should be negotiated at your first meeting. Children should be encouraged to think about whether details of dreams and what comes up in the group should be confidential. Maybe some members will say when they especially want personal information kept within the group. Whatever you negotiate about confidentiality, remember that dreams can elicit emotive, previously undisclosed material, and the climate of unbroken trust is vital in such a sensitive area. Clearly, you need to take into account child protection issues, which include the revelation of abuse, and you need to be aware of guidelines that assure the best interests of the child. So if you are running a group in a school or residential setting, for instance, find out what the code is regarding confidentiality.

Establish ground rules

It is useful to go through this aspect with the children. At the first meeting when you have begun to set the atmosphere as one which is about having fun and learning by sharing with one another, ask the children how you as a group can best work together. Encourage open discussion and ensure everyone has a chance to say what he or she wants. Be guided by your group. In my own experience of working with groups the following ground rules work well:

- We will listen whenever a person is talking.
- We will try to understand how he or she feels about the dream and not make fun or be unkind.
- We will share our ideas to help each other.
- We will be honest.
- We will work together.
- We will use the phrase 'If this were my dream, I would…' to explore another person's dream rather than saying 'Your dream means…'.

Create the right atmosphere

A dream group should feel warm, comfortable, caring, supportive and positive. Children will feel confident when they are a valued part of the group and will flourish in a place they enjoy. Successful groups are ones which are run on ethical lines where no child feels exploited and every one's voice is heard.

> 'I don't tell anyone my dreams, I always think they are going to laugh at me.'
>
> Jack (9)

Everyone can participate

There are no right or wrong interpretations about dreams. There is no list that will definitively tell you what each dream means. The dream belongs to the dreamer and dream sharing helps that dreamer to understand the message for herself. So encourage everyone to join in the discussion and to listen to various points of view while ensuring that everyone understands that an explanation or interpretation needs to feel right, to resonate for the dreamer, before it should be taken on board.

Children can take it in turns in the group to present a dream. This can be done by talking about it or by drawing it. In the latter case a shy child might want to show the drawing to the group and answer questions about the dream activity, rather than giving a long explanation. Be sensitive to the level of confidence of the child and always help as much as you can to bring out those children who feel ill at ease in a group.

Find a creative approach for the group

Groups are dynamic organisms, they flow and change. With this in mind find an approach that works best with your group. For instance, some dream groups run well when at each meeting every person has some time to talk about a dream they have had in the previous week. In this way each person has some time at each meeting. However, this might not suit every-one's needs.

Another approach is for the group to decide to work in depth on one or two dreams. This can be useful if someone has had a particularly disturbing dream and wants to help in unravelling its meaning.

A third method is a more structured, thematic approach. You decide what areas of dreams you want to work on or learn about and spend a session on each. So you might devise a programme to include animals in dreams, dream monsters, nightmares, and problem-solving in dreams, and so on. In each case, encourage the children to consult their own dream records for relevant material, and see if you can find illustrations – pictures, postcards, artwork – to bring to the group.

Dream records

Encourage each child to keep a record of his dreams in a special notebook. Drawings too will form part of this dream history, and every dream should be dated. Over time a pattern may emerge which will help the dreamer identify the 'message' of the dream.

At the last session of a dream group it is helpful to look at the develop-ments that have taken place by having a kind of 'retrospective exhibition'.

Sharing in the rewards of growth as well as being part of the process leaves everyone feeling positive.

The role of facilitator

I use the word facilitator rather than leader because the former is one who helps in the process, whereas a leader usually has a much more directive role. The exciting aspect of dream-work is that we never know quite where dreams will lead us, and during an exploration of a dream, insights can come from anyone.

Your role as facilitator is to provide the setting and do most of the organisation, and then to be a kind of conductor of the music, holding the players together to achieve the best interpretation for the dream creator. The dreamer is the composer, and ultimately it is to provide a satisfactory expression of her creation that we join together. Along the way all members of the group have a chance to play, to learn and to enjoy the process and production.

Be tender – in sharing dreams we share our deepest selves.

A practical guide for working with children's dreams

How do you console your child after a nightmare? What can you do to tame dream monsters? Whether you are a caring parent whose child has a bad dream or a person who works with children as a nurse, teacher, child-minder or youth worker, there are times when you will want to 'do something' to help. This guide gives you a set of simple techniques to help you work with dreams and nightmares. Should you try these and problems with dreams do not diminish, then seek professional help.

- Try to create a caring, accepting, non-judgemental atmosphere. Dreams are not 'right' or 'wrong', so please don't tell a child that they are bad, silly or horrible to dream whatever they have dreamt about.

- Respect the child's need for confidentiality. If she chooses to talk to other people about her dreams – fine; but do not abuse the trust she has put in you by talking to others without her permission.

- Listen to what the child says and ask open questions that encourage her to explore the dream. For example, 'How did you feel in the dream?', 'What helped you when you were being chased?', 'What was the nicest part of the fairyland place you went to?' By listening you show the child that you value what she has to say and this increases the child's self-esteem and trust in you. Dreams cannot be worked on unless there is trust between the dream teller and the dream hearer; this alliance is a vital part of the process.

- Allow the child to express her feelings about the dream and go at her own pace. Do not force a child to go on talking about dreams when she wants to stop. Respect her right to privacy, remembering that you are not a psychoanalyst, but a supportive adult in a non-clinical setting. Most children need a grown-up friend, not a therapist.

- Help the child make links to events in waking life. If a child has an upsetting dream, gently try to find out if there is anything bothering her in waking life. Children can become much more aware of internal psychic pressures by working on dreams. Carl's dream described below gives an example of this developing self-awareness.

- Some children believe that if they talk about a dream it will come true. Help educate children about dreams so that they understand the purpose of dreaming.

- If the child wants to, and it seems appropriate, encourage more active ways of working on dreams:
  - Draw the dream. Look at it. Talk about it. Ask the child if she would like to change it and if so how? She might want her dog to come and be with her, so let her draw in her dog. She might want the offending monster to be destroyed so let her paint over it or cut it out. The aim is to generate positive responses to dealing with whatever has caused the distress.
  - Act out the dream. If the child has been chased in the dream, she may, with your help, feel secure enough to

re-enact the dream. You might have to play a chasing monster; but before you start, plan a way for the child to deal successfully with the threat. Maybe she can make friends with it; maybe she wants to destroy it; perhaps she could talk to it and tell it to stop being so horrible. The aim is to enable the child to confront the danger and, with your support, to find a way of dealing with that dream situation.

Carl (9) has temper tantrums in which he directs much of his anger against his mother. One evening, after a particularly aggressive outburst, his mother sent him to bed. That night Carl had a nightmare:

> 'There was an eye running about and a devil killed me, but I came back alive and killed my mum because the devil was controlling me.'

He woke up with a pencil in his hand, held like a dagger. This sort of dream lets the child express the anger and frustration felt during waking hours. The highly dramatised dream drama also enabled Carl to deny his responsibility, since it is the devil in the dream who is 'controlling' him. We all find it difficult to accept intense negative emotions that we feel, and Carl is no different from many adults and children. He does not really want to own the 'bad' part of himself.

So, what can we do to help youngsters like Carl grow through such feelings? One thing is to talk about the dream and talk about the feelings, reassuring him that all of us have 'good' and 'bad' feelings, that we all at times want to hit back at people who we think have hurt us and let us down. Explain that part of growing up is learning to control the impulses to attack others. Dreams let us express those hostile feelings without physically hurting the person they are aimed at. Carl can get his own back on his mother but still wake up caring for her – and with a sense of relief that she is unharmed!

Such violent dreams are not particularly unusual, especially where there are a lot of conflicts in a very close relationship. Whatever the cause, these dreams can act as a catharsis and a starting point for talking through unresolved feelings of distress and unhappiness. Carl said he does tell his mother about his dreams, so they would be an ideal vehicle for them to talk about their life together. He also needs to be reassured that he is not 'mad' or going to be a criminal because he has these dreams. He needs to know that almost all children and adults have disturbing dreams about which they feel anxious or ashamed.

Marie (8) had a particularly traumatic time when her brother suffered a deep head wound. She regularly dreams that this happens again and, most terrifyingly, that it is her father who hit him in the first place. In other dreams she and her brother are locked up by a man who is jealous of them, and he is going to kill them. In her happiest dream she saved someone because she was changed into 'Supergirl'. She has to become like Wonder Woman in order to protect others! But who is protecting her? Her dreams certainly indicate that no obvious person fulfils that role.

Marie hoped that my book might help children to forget about their dreams because all her dreams do is scare her. What I hope my book will do is not help children to 'forget' dreams but enable parents and others who care for and work with children to realise that children's deepest fears and anxieties signal to us through dreams. We as responsible caring adults can help them work through the pain and terror. We need to show them we care enough to listen.

Gideon (10) recalled a recurring dream in which he was inescapably entwined in a massive black metallic structure. He said, looking back, that it represented his life at that age. This imagery of being enclosed, trapped, held in impersonal surroundings and being powerless, figures in many children's dreams. You can help a child to make links with waking circumstances. Where does he feel trapped and why? You may be able to highlight an escape route that he has not noticed.

Hannah (12), a happy successful extrovert, describes her dreams as usually connected to the daily events of her life. However, just now and then she has a typical 'chase' dream:

> 'Someone is running after me and no matter how fast I run the other person is always gaining on me but never catches me.'

The sense of frustration at not making progress is there, but Hannah succeeds in avoiding the threat that pursues her. This is a healthy sign; when young people talk about such dreams, point out such positive aspects.

One final point here – children need information about the physical effects of dreams. In particular, boys should be told about nocturnal ejaculation, 'wet dreams'. A wet dream for a boy who has not been told about such events is frightening. While few boys talk of night-time ejaculation related to dreams, this is to do with embarrassment about sex rather than an absence of such dreams. Explain to children that wet dreams are a normal part of growing up, they are part of the way in which the body is getting ready for mature sexual activity.

I sometimes use prepared 'Dream Times' worksheets when working with children. I have included a couple here to give you an idea of what they are. If you want any further material please contact me at the address at the end of the book.

Dream Communications

The Talmud, an important guide for Jewish people, says

'An uninterpreted dream is like an unopened letter.'

In other words if you don't pay attention to your dreams it is like receiving a letter but not bothering to read it. You can miss some important information that way!

- Think about a dream that you have had and do a drawing of it in the box.

- Give it a title: ....

- What do you think this dream was trying to communicate to you? What message did this 'dream letter' want to deliver to you?.............................
....
....

Dream Explorer

Some people think that the dreamer makes every part of the dream because it has something to tell the dreamer.

This is like being a film producer or director, you choose the script, the actors, the setting, the dialogue and the action. So, when looking at your dream use the Dream Explorer to help you explore it.

You are the dream director, so first of all –

Give your dream a title.

Imagine your dream was a film and answer these questions.

- Who are the most important actors?

- Where is the dream set?

- What is special about this dream setting?

- What is the atmosphere like? E.g. scary, calm?

- Is there anything you want to change in it?

- What is the message of your dream?

Harry Potter Dreaming

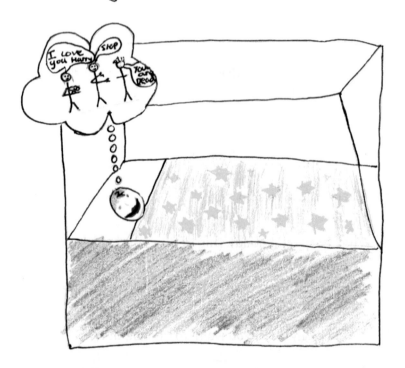

Harry Potter Dreaming

Chapter Four

A Short Introduction
to the Dreams of Harry Potter

Harry Potter, the world-famous hero of J.K. Rowling's award-winning series, has a number of highly significant dreams. Many prepare him for future events whilst others connect him to his earliest trauma when his parents were killed.

In the first book *Harry Potter and the Philosopher's Stone*, Harry dreams about a flying motorbike. He has no conscious memory of when he was a baby and the giant Hagrid took him away after the attack on his parents. Through the night sky the baby was transported to the strange world of 'Muggles', those people without magical powers. His dreams reconnect him to earlier events even though he has no waking recall of them.

Harry hated living with the despicable Dursleys, his only living relatives, and, like many children who are unhappy, he dreamed of an unknown relation coming to take him away to a better home. Also in *The Philosopher's Stone* is the dream where Harry wears the turban of one of his teachers, Professor Quirrell. From within the turban a voice tells him he must switch to Slytherin House because that is his destiny. The turban gets heavier and tighter, crushing his head, and all the while his hated fellow pupil Malfoy looks on. Malfoy changes into the equally hated teacher

Snape, who laughs at his distress. At the end of the dream a burst of green light wakes him up.

This example of shapeshifting, when Malfoy morphs into Snape, shows how Harry links them together. He knows they are connected in some way, which we learn about as the stories develop. Also, the green light, though he does not recall it on waking, is the light that appeared when he was almost killed by Lord Voldemort. Harry had recurring nightmares about his parents disappearing in a flash of green light as a high-pitched voice laughed. These can be seen as typical post-traumatic stress dreams where the original event is repeated. Interestingly, Harry finds that they are less frequent when he is physically worn out after Quidditch training.

In *Harry Potter and the Chamber of Secrets* he dreams that he is on show in a zoo. On the cage is a sign, 'Under-age Wizard', and people stare at him as he lies on a bed of straw. He sees the house elf, Dobby, and pleads for help, but Dobby tells him he is safe there. The dream reveals his feeling of being trapped by the Dursleys who hate him yet have to let him live with them, but also his fears of being under attack from the dark side. They also forewarn him of the role Dobby will play in his future.

This dream also shows how Harry is affected by the fact that he is the most famous boy wizard in the world. This is a mixed blessing: he really wants to be an ordinary boy but destiny has given him a hero's journey, a mythic quest with all the obstacles and unexpected challenges which mark such a journey.

As Harry starts the new term in *The Prisoner of Azkaban*, his dreams show a deeper connection to his dead mother. In one awful nightmare, illustrated in Sonia's picture at the start of this chapter, clammy, rotting hands appear and he hears his mother's terrified voice pleading with Voldemort to spare her son. When he wakes he realises that his mother gave up her own life to protect him. This revelation, this awareness, sad as it is, lets him know how much he was loved. For many children, dreaming of those who have died can be a great comfort, though tinged with sorrow too.

The magical elements of these stories weave through Harry's dreams. In another he is walking through a forest when he finds himself following something silvery white. He can't see it clearly but he knows he must catch up with it. The speed of both Harry and the light increases then he hears the pounding of hooves, and just as he reaches a clearing he is woken up by a commotion in the dormitory. The silvery white and the hooves are important as we discover towards the end of the third book in the series. These link him both to his father and his own powers as a wizard, but I won't tell you why just in case you've not read it yet. It might help to know that the stag is an ancient symbol of renewal as it sheds its horns and regrows them.

Harry's dream themes are typical of so many children's. He dreams of falling, of being chased by Malfoy's gang, of fire and of being attacked. Before an important Quidditch match he dreams he has overslept, that the other team sit astride fire-breathing dragons and that he's forgotten to bring his own Firebolt to ride on. Anxiety themes that children would easily identify with.

Dreams continue to play an important role in *Harry Potter and the Goblet of Fire.* They bring him closer and closer to the events that marked him with his lightning-shaped scar. They introduce him to the full horror of Voldemort. By this time Harry is now fourteen; he sometimes does not tell others about his anxious dreams in case it makes him seem as if he is too worried. This self-censorship is quite usual at this age. However, he understands now that his dreams alert him to the presence of his would-be destroyer Voldemort, and he asks others what he should do. Harry also learns that as we sleep our mind continues to work on what is worrying us and one morning he wakes up with a fully formed plan that will protect his godfather Sirius Black.

In one chapter of *The Goblet of Fire* called 'The Dream' Harry flies on the back of an eagle owl and lands in a deserted house in which is a dark room. He meets a huge snake, Lord Voldemort and his servant Wormtail and hears the plan that he is to be killed. Harry learns he is to be fed to the snake. Once more his dream warns him of the danger that stalks him and expresses his deep anxiety. It also triggers a physical reaction – his scar hurts. This physical response to disturbing dreams happens with some children who feel fear. Harry does talk with his closest friends, but others who feel less connected may keep their anxiety hidden. As in Harry's case physical pain can arise in such children when they recognise, on an unconscious level, that they are in grave danger.

All in all, the dreams of Harry Potter reflect the emotional world of children, the symbolic power of the unconscious, and show how dreams can reveal events that have been hidden from waking knowledge. Sometimes our dreams are far wiser than we know, and for anyone who wants to help children understand their dreams, the dreams of brave Harry Potter might be a good place to start.

PART TWO
Dream Themes

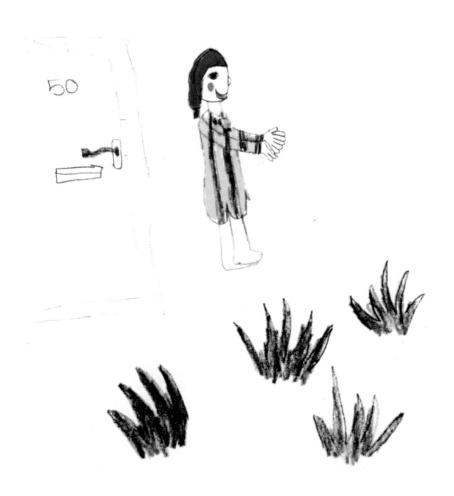

Walking in Our Dreams

Chapter Five

Welcome to the Dreaming

We may expect to find in dreams everything that has ever been of
significance in the life of humanity.
Carl Gustav Jung in Anthony Stevens' *Private Myths*

From Aborigines to Native Americans, from Vikings to present day
eco-warriors, dreams have played a role in the cultural life of the community. We share this world of dreams with animals – it is easy to see as they
twitch and growl in their sleep. I was fascinated to learn in a recent newspaper report that further proof is available: a gorilla that had been taught
sign language, put two signs together to form the word sleep pictures,
probably to indicate the visual part of his sleep life.

Layers of dreaming

Dreams belong to the individual child, but they go far beyond this because
in dreams we find layers of meaning and connection. The first layer is the
personal, unique experience of the child, the second is the layer that relates
to his immediate environment, the next is to the wider world and
world-wide issues, and the last layer, which Jung called the collective
unconscious, is the one that connects him to all that has gone before. It acts
as the storehouse of myths and symbols to which everyone has access and
it is the source of myths in all societies.

The American psychologist Sharon Saline describes a dream that demonstrates the idea that dreams connect us to our ancient ancestors. She cites the interesting dream of a 9-year-old girl. The girl is with her friend jumping on her bed. Rings appeared and they jumped with these using them as monkey bars, and as they did so, 'With every swing we went through a picture of a generation of our family until we got to the pilgrimage…'. The dream portrays her present life with her friend, and her ancestors who came to America as pilgrims. She understood through her 'dream procession' that she is carrying the family forward to future generations.

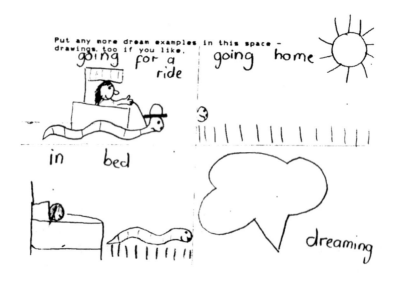

Girl and Caterpillar

Dreaming traditions

Throughout history, groups have used dreams for the good of both the individual and the group. In many ancient traditions we find that dreams are seen as the mechanism where past and future can be accessed and where men might meet gods. It helps children to value their own dream life when they understand how dreams are used by different groups. So we will now see what others have done.

British anthropologist Hugh Brody, in his magnificent book *The Other side of Eden: Hunter-gatherers, Farmers and the Shaping of the World*, describes how dreams still play a central role in a respectful relationship with the earth and the animals who walk on it. He says of the Dunne-za hunters: 'To find animals that are willing to be killed [they] travel along trails that reveal themselves in dreams. How else can they travel such distances; how else process such huge quantities of data; how otherwise make decisions … Dreaming is the mind's way of combining and using more information than the conscious mind can hold.'

Australian Aborigines

Dreaming is of vital importance in aboriginal traditions. For Australian Aborigines dreaming is a symbol of their heroic past, which has to be re-enacted in order to keep it alive. Without the dreaming, they say, we are lost. They also believe that life and death are part of a cycle that begins and ends in dream-time and that during the experience of dreaming we are freed from the limitations of time and space.

Aborigines believe that dreams reveal events from the distant past and the future, through the myths that come in dreams or via dead ancestors who come in dreams. The dreams are so important to Australian Aborigines that they do not make a strong distinction between waking reality and dream events. There are variations between the different tribal groups.

The Narranga-ga tribe say that the human spirit can leave the dreamer's body and wander about and make contact with other spirits or with the spirits of dead people. The Jupagalk believe that a person who is sick can be helped by a dream visit of a dead relative. This view is found throughout the world and by children too. Certainly, British children told me about dreams in which a dead relative, such as a grandmother, has helped them when they were ill – more of this in Chapter 5.

Animals are important in Aboriginal dreams as they signify a guide or totem which comes to help the dreamer. The importance of dream animals as power guides is common in many native traditions, as we will see with Native Americans.

Native American

> Many North American Indian tribes...attach great significance to dreams. Of special significance...were guardian spirit dreams... the Plains Indian youth...will deliberately detach himself from the group, fast in seclusion, and await the response of his guardian spirit in his dreams.
>
> Carl W. O'Neill, *Dreams, Culture, and the Individual*

There are many tribes of Native American Indians, each with its own unique tradition. Dreams play a significant role, particularly in dream sharing where the community gets together to talk about individual dreams that may hold particular information for them all. The Hopi believe that good dreams are held in the heart but bad dreams must be talked about and the problems they bring to light must be worked on and resolved.

In the Shasta tribe the first sign that someone might have shamanic power comes when they dream of a dead ancestor, and many believe initiatory dreams come in childhood. Dream animals again, are seen as power guides or guardian spirits.

The Iroquois have a theory known as 'soul-wish-manifesting'. They believe that human beings have souls that have a concealed inborn desire, which is stored at our deepest level. The purpose of dreams is to make these deep desires known, so the Iroquois record their dreams; they try to interpret what their soul wants and use dream specialists to interpret the dreams correctly.

The Mistassini Cree live in Quebec and are a subarctic people who exist by hunting and trapping. Like so many other nomadic groups who live in close harmony with their land, they use divinatory dreams to help with their hunt. They also see them as important for creativity and spiritual guidance. The anthropologist Adrian Tanner in his book *Bringing Home Animals* explains how power is believed to be brought to the Cree in dreams, where they learn special songs, techniques for making and decorating their clothes and shamanistic healing techniques.

Shamans

> The most powerful Dunne-za dreamers, when they learned the Christian story of the afterlife, reported that they had found routes to heaven. This was a shamanic response to missionary ideas; if there was a trail to be discovered, the dreamer must find it.
>
> Hugh Brody, *The Other Side of Eden*

The word shaman originated in Siberia and is another word for medicine man or woman. These priests or healers use dreams as part of their spiritual development. Shamanism is based on the belief that good and evil spirits pervade our world and that these spirits can be influenced by those who have Shamanic power. In altered states of consciousness and in dreams the shaman makes contact with these spirits and brings back information for his community. He also uses dreams to diagnose illness and to find out how to treat a sick person, what herbs to use, and so on.

A shaman is also a seer in the dark and can 'shapeshift', or change his shape, in order to travel between worlds. Disguise or taking on the character of animals or ancestors is part of the waking process too. Shaman masks are sometimes made in the shape of a zigzag to represent a flash of lightning. This symbolises the shaman's ability to move between the heavenly and earthly worlds. I wonder if this inspired J.K. Rowling, the author of the Harry Potter series, to provide Harry with the zigzag scar he has on his forehead?

China

Dreams have always been significant for the Chinese. They had dream incubation temples, as did the Ancient Greeks. In these sacred temples a person would go to 'incubate', to bring about, a dream which answered a specific question or which gave guidance to the dreamer. Up to the 16th century, all government officials had to go to a dream temple to receive guidance before making official declarations or introducing any new political policy. As with so many other cultures, the Chinese believed that the spiritual soul, which has the same shape as the physical body, could travel to other realms and visit other souls during sleep.

The famous philosopher Confucius once dreamt that he was a butter-fly. When he woke up he asked himself if he was a man dreaming he was a butterfly, or a butterfly dreaming he was a man! This dream is often referred to when people are discussing the reality of the world we experi-ence. Certainly, children often feel their dreams are just as 'real' as their waking experiences and sometimes confuse them as Catherine described at the end of Chapter 1.

Universal connections

There are universal dream themes, which include falling, being naked, being chased, being lost and there are universal dream symbols such as water, the sun, caves and houses. The dream of Danielle (7) seems to connect to the earliest phase of human development, before human beings emerged from our watery origin:

> 'I was walking on the waves of an ocean, then lived in the water and blew bubbles like a fish.'

While Danielle was happy in her dream, fish and animals often symbolise threatening forces in the dreams of children. They may represent arche-typal elements in the Jungian sense, in that they are not based on personal experience, but stem from our common human heritage, our collective unconscious memory of the past. There was a time in our evolutionary history when animals and insects were daily enemies, and for young children fear of raw animal potency is apparent in dreams.

Yvette (13) from New Jersey told me of a dream which echoes this watery connection:

> 'There was a dark space around me. It was warm and comfortable. A huge monster, a fish/dragon ate me up. It swallowed me up whole and I can remember my stomach doing a flip-flop.'

Dreams of time and place

> 'I dreamed I was kidnapped at school and left to die.'
>
> Victoria (10)

In the collection of dreams gathered by Charles Kimmins in 1918, I could find no references to dreams of being kidnapped recorded for the 2–13 age group. There are so many similar themes in other areas, yet children then did not report fear dreams of kidnapping. How is this explained? Is it a reflection of our society in which children feel unprotected? Is it that the influence of media and its content ensures that few children feel completely safe? Whatever the causes, these dreams tell us that many of our children do not feel safe. Finn (7) from a remote farming community in County Tyrone in Ireland has the ubiquitous dreams of ghosts and says that he has never had a happy dream, a frequent lament from children. Finn drew me a picture of an evil-looking man who was a kidnapper; he took Finn away in a bag. In Finn's drawing there is a sad-looking figure, all scrunched in a bag swung over the villain's shoulder; from the bag came a bubble of sound, plaintively saying 'help!' Threatening dream characters change from monsters and ghosts to anonymous males and impersonal enemies or, worse, known members of the family.

Cities bring their own share of dangers. Dean (10) dreams of being beaten up, someone coming upstairs to get him, and monsters. He said, quite candidly: 'If I watch scary videos, I have nightmares.' He also, occasionally now, has dreams of riding his bike and being knocked off it again. Two years before, he was hit by a car while out in the street riding and he was in hospital for some time with a broken leg. In his dreams he relives the trauma as his mind tries to find a way of making sense of the experience. Until Dean comes to terms with the shock, his accident dream will probably continue. If he can talk through the feelings he had at the time of the accident, his fears and even maybe his feeling of guilt at being in some way to blame, then the dream will probably go away. Until the trauma is exorcised the dream will keep nudging him to finish off the 'unfinished business'.

Gloria (13), from London, recognises the fear of the streets shared by many women, young and old alike. She described one dream:

> 'I was walking alone in town and a man grabbed me and he raped and stabbed me. It was really horrible.'

Though this dream terrified her she still felt that the worst dream she had ever had was one in which her mother left her.

Ghosts and monsters

I met Ben (6) when I went to visit some travelling families in their caravan homes. Ben shares a small caravan with his nine brothers and sisters and his mother and father and his dreams reflect his Irish origin:

> 'There was a Banshee on top of the roof. It flew into the room and got a girl, cut her up and made her into stew.'

Neither of Ben's parents could read or write, and most of the children had spent little time in school owing to their nomadic life and because of the hostility made plain by settled communities. However, most of their traditional stories are passed on orally, and you can see that tales heard at home are highly influential:

> 'I dreamt of a headless man riding a horse, and once, when we pulled into a graveyard to stay the night, I dreamt of ghosts and things coming for me.'

Whatever the age, the feeling of being under threat from impersonal enemies is palpable, so while Saima (7) dreams of 'witches taking me away from my mum and dad', and 'white ghosts' who tell her that her mother and father are dead, Barry (13) dreamt:

> 'There were flashing lights outside my window and when I looked out people were running everywhere. People were getting killed all over the place and when I looked closer I saw myself down there running around and hiding.'

Developmental stress, unpleasant events or trauma and general everyday unhappiness are revealed in the manifest content of the dreams of ordinary children. In a way this should be no surprise, as children have to undergo such major developmental changes as they mature, and the mastery of these emotional and physical changes is the work of childhood. Dreams often communicate just how difficult such work is, a fact we adults all too frequently overlook.

Houses as symbols

When I was researching my book *Women Dreaming* I soon realised that in the majority of women's dreams the recurring image of the house symbolised the person's sense of themselves. Different levels of the house may be used to represent distinctive psychological aspects. So the attic may symbolise the thinking processes, being in our 'heads'; the cellars may signify being in touch with our unconscious, dark hidden drives; and so on. When I came across Helen's (13) dream, which she had at 9 years of age, it became obvious that this can be a potent symbol early in our lives. Helen dreamt:

> 'The house fell down. It fell down in stages. First the front, then the back, then the middle. My father, sister and I were all in the house but my mum was out at work. We were trying to burrow under the floor to get out of the way of falling bricks, and all I could think about was what Mum would think when she got in.'

On a very simple level Helen might be worried about her mother's reaction when she comes home from work and finds the house a shambles, so Helen's dream may be dramatically depicting that scenario. However, it may reveal that Helen feels her defences, as symbolised by the protective structure of the house, are falling apart. Her father and sister are affected by this also and are equally trying to avoid the danger, but they need to go deeper in order to escape. What does Helen's family have to dig or delve into to resolve the situation?

Dreams can influence whole communities, either directly or indirectly. As described by French writer Raymond de Becker in *The Understanding of Dreams,* the Second World War might never have happened if a key character had not had a life-saving dream. During the First World War a German corporal fell asleep in his bunker in the front lines. He had a startling dream that an artillery shell made a direct hit on the bunker in which he was sleeping. He woke up and ran away from the bunker, which was immediately destroyed by an artillery shell. That man was Adolf Hitler. He believed his dream had saved his life and given him a sign to set out and change the world; he felt invincible.

Children's fears

Fear of not achieving well in school, being suspected of lying, poor school reports and being sent to the headteacher, all figured highly in children's rating of stressful life events in a cross-cultural study of children from six countries published in 1987 in the journal *Child Psychology and Psychiatry* (by Yamamoto and colleagues). They felt acutely the humiliation meted out by sarcastic teachers. What the children said they felt was often different from what adults around perceived, indicating that we must listen to what children tell us rather than assume we know how they feel. We need to try to understand the structure and function of childhood from the inside and one way is to attend to what children communicate through dreams.

The wider world affects school life and details are regularly included in dreams. Kimberley (11) relates:

> 'I was in my classroom alone, nobody was there. I heard a helicopter flying around outside, then it dropped a pink-wrapped present with a purple-and-yellow bow. I picked up the present and untied it and bang! Then the whole school blows up and I die and go to hell!'

At some level Kimberley recognises that she is in an explosive situation, as she was in her Belfast home, where helicopters patrolled day and night. However, it may well relate to another situation that on the surface is quite pleasant and nicely wrapped up, but blows up in her face. When you meet a dream like this help the child to play with the language and ideas. Does she feel that something is about to blow up? Has anyone said to her 'Go to hell'?

Emma (10), who lives with her mother and three sisters, has many nightmares. In this one she goes to the rescue:

> 'I had a nightmare of my sister falling off a high cliff and I jumped after her but at the bottom of the cliff a man walked to where my sister was going to fall and just caught her and I felt myself bang on the floor and woke up.'

Fortunately there is an adult figure who can successfully intervene where her efforts fail. The sensation of falling out of bed is incorporated into the dream here. This is not at all unusual as we noted earlier.

Dreaming in the new millennium

All around the world there is an upsurge of interest in dreams and dreaming. In psychotherapy, in holistic medicine, in personal development and in studies of creativity and problem-solving, dreams play a significant role. They also reflect our cultural heritage. Chicago-based dream researcher Anthony Shafton in a 1999 article in *Dream Time* shows how prophetic dreaming was taken for granted by African-Americans in the days of slavery. Now in the general population of America between 25 and 50 per cent believe in precognitive dreams, while 92 per cent of the black African-Americans he interviewed did so. This obviously has implications for the way children view their dreams, so we need to be mindful of cultural differences when they talk of their dreams.

As children learn more about the problems that beset our planet – pollution, climate change, globalisation, and so on – their dreams reflect anxiety. They speak of dreams in which the world ends, tidal waves destroy cities and disasters strike randomly. Douglas (9) dreamt about the ozone layer breaking up and the heat on earth becoming unbearable. He also has frightening dreams about nuclear war. He said: 'Children just learn these adult problems and think it's not very nice, and then dream about them.'

Both boys and girls dream of danger from outside forces such as fire, and these dreams increase after the age of 8. Chantelle (9) has an amalgamation of fears: being shot in the back, her family being imprisoned in a dungeon and the shadows in her room. In her happiest dream she finds a way to erase all this fear by 'killing the devil and making things better for the world and for me'.

Dreaming has relevance for children whether they live in hunter-gatherer tribes in Canada or communities in London. In the next chapter we will explore the significance of nightmares that trouble our children.

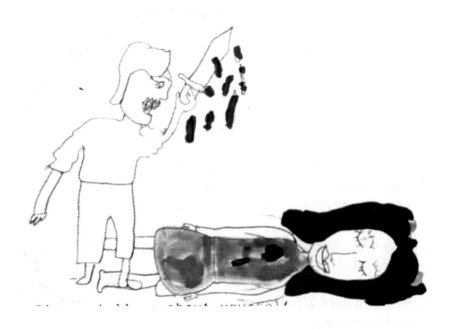

He Killed Me

Chapter Six

Nightmare Taming

Parents do not know what they do when they leave tender babes
alone to go to sleep in the dark...
                Charles Lamb in Walter de la Mare's *Behold, This Dreamer*

The English essayist and critic Charles Lamb (1775–1834) was plagued
by nightmares as a child. As Walter de la Mare describes in *Behold, This
Dreamer*, Lamb said: 'The night-time solitude, and the dark, were my hell.'
Children today also share his fear of the dark and worry about what sleep
may bring, so in this chapter we will look at how to help children banish
nightmares.

> 'If I am upset or angry about something, then I have horrible,
> frightening dreams which ends up in me sitting up in bed and
> feeling very scared.'
>
> Alice (12)

The word nightmare originates from *night* plus the Old English word *mære*
meaning an evil spirit. Nightmares usually occur in REM sleep during the
latter part of the night, when all types of dreaming are most common. You
can recognise nightmares by the way in which the child wakes up in tears,
or complains that in his 'bad dream' he has been chased, attacked or had
some kind of catastrophe. With gentle reassurance the child usually returns
to sleep.

Nightmares do have a positive role. They are part of our early warning system. They warn of turbulence below a calm exterior. We might feel that our children are doing fine, they seem happy enough, yet nightmares tell us otherwise. Whether caused by school yard squabbles or disturbance within the family, they are distress signals to alert us to action.

Typical nightmare themes

Fear of separation

Part of the process of growing up is learning to become independent, to separate. This can be a frightening experience, and it shows up in children's dreams. Typically it is revealed in themes of being lost, kidnapped or abandoned. Ten-year-old Dean used to have this dream when he was about 6:

> 'I used to be out in the garden, in the dark, and this bus used to come along and pick me up with all these other people in it. Then they took me underground to all these caverns where all these witches used to scare me and little men used to be really nasty to me. The bus would come and take me home again but it was horrible.'

We can see how the dream reflects anxiety about being 'taken away', being separated from people who care for him and being at the mercy of evil 'witches'. For young children witches, like monsters, symbolise powerful forces that can hurt. They also express a child's fear that there are some things in their world over which they have no control. As parents we need to reassure children that we will protect them and that, though there are dangers in the world, we can and will be there to take care of them until they are big enough to look after themselves.

> 'The most frightening dream I ever had was when I got lost and while I was away I found out that my mother and grandmother had died so I never went home and a fierce dog killed me.'
>
> Cathy (10)

Often children fantasise that when they are away from home something bad will happen. This is particularly the case where there has been some form of family trauma, such as a divorce or bereavement. In fact, some children actively express this by refusing to go to school. As I say in *Helping Children to Manage Loss*, the child may not be consciously aware of this fear, but at a deep level they need to stay with the remaining parent to ensure that the bad thing does not happen to him or her. Cathy's dream is a good example of such fears.

> 'I often dream that I am in a crowded village, in the nude. I can see my friends and family. I see my enemies round me closing in and my family and friends are walking away. Just as the bad things close in the ground breaks and I fall down, down, down. I see a light getting bigger and bigger. Then I wake, usually about two in the morning.'
>
> Adrian (12)

Falling and being naked are universal themes. Adrian's insecurity as he moves towards adolescence, away from childhood dependency, is mirrored in the dream images. I wonder if Adrian was born at 2am? Midwives and others who work with babies have told me that they notice children are often fretful about the same hour that they were born, as if recalling the birth trauma.

Stress is a factor in causing both nightmares and night terrors. Psychiatrist Irwin Knopf has suggested that very sensitive children are more prone to nightmares, while those who suffer night terrors may have an immature nervous system. Generally nightmares and night terrors do not require medical treatment, as they stop spontaneously. If they happen to your child your reassurance is needed. Listen to what the child has to say, and sensitively respond to fears that are voiced. Also consider the daily events of the child: Is he experiencing unusual stress at school or home? Has he had a change, such as moving house or being ill, which has upset him? Children do not always speak to us of their concerns; often they communicate distress by changes in behaviour, bed-wetting, or regressing to an earlier stage.

Being abandoned

In their nightmares children dream that they are abandoned by the people who are supposed to take care of them. This may include the ultimate fear which is that their parents will die and they will be left with no one.

> 'The most frightening dream I have had is that all my family die.'
>
> Tim (10)

It is hard for children to talk to parents about death yet they do think about it and the fears are expressed in dreams. There are all sorts of situations in which children's fears of being left are expressed. Adam (9) had this dream after his mother had taken him to a new church where there was a separate Bible class for children.

> 'I used to have this dream again and again. In it my mum took me to a church and up the stairs and left me. Then this wizard used to be there boiling up a cauldron. There was a cage in the corner and he used to try and get me in there.'

The dream is like the story of Hansel and Gretel who are locked in a cage until the witch fattens them up. His dream links to his fear of being abandoned. Adam told me that he found the church a 'bit spooky and weird', though he had never told his mother about his feelings – or his dreams.

In helping children to express their fears, fairy-tales can be very helpful. For centuries fairy-tales were the main source of entertainment for children. One reason why they are so potent, as Bruno Bettelheim, one of the greatest child psychologists of the 20th century, so lucidly explains in *The Uses of Enchantment* (which I consider the most insightful book about fairy-stories ever written), is that so many express the abandonment children feel in everyday situations: when they are left at nursery, when they are put to bed, even when parents go out and a well-liked baby-sitter is left in charge. Feelings of being deserted may be quite powerful. However, working through such feelings, surviving them and feeling all right, leads to liberation and independence. In many books it is only after children have been left, lost or abandoned that things really start happening for them, as it does for Harry Potter. The central characters discover new worlds and new capabilities previously hidden from themselves, and begin to grasp the fact that they can separate from their parents and become autonomous.

Bettelheim shows how important it is that children do not experience only pleasant, wish-fulfilling, happy fairy-stories: a balance is needed. Children feel anger and hostility, violent emotion and feelings of helplessness and fairy-stories enable them to realise they are not alone, that others have such feelings and living involves a struggle between good and bad, fortune and misfortune. Fairy-tales appeal to both sides of reality and help children deal with their own deep, inner conflicts. Often dreams have a fairy-tale quality about them and you can help children work through nightmares by making this connection.

Mythological themes of devouring are universal, as psychoanalysts Jung and Fordham point out. In the first half of 10-year-old Zania's dream a lovely, old woman was so kind to her that eventually she accepted an offer to tea. Of course, once she got to the lady's house the trouble started:

> 'She locked the door and hid the key. I said, "What are you doing?" "Oh, nothing," she said. Then she told me to sit down and after I sat down she seemed to do something behind me. When I looked round I saw a horrible face. It was the old woman. She was really a witch. Then she said to me, "My name is Zelda and I hate children. I brought you here because I want to pull your skin off like the other children and now it's your turn." I shouted but it was no use, she came up closer and closer then suddenly I woke up.'

Helping children manage their fears means helping them to realise they are not powerless victims, unable to affect change. Fairy-tales show that the weak are not always overcome: wit and persistence, honesty and willingness to confront danger may still win the day. You can help children by talking through fears at the once-removed position. So, we could say to Zania: 'What could you do if you were in a room and someone locked you in?' Then look at possible solutions – climb out of the window? Shout for help? Pretend someone was waiting outside for you? Share your ideas with your child. and let her know you empathise. You can also use this technique with fairy-tales. What else could Goldilocks do to find a place to eat? Working towards solutions influences the mind-set of the child so she becomes more confident and solution-focused, rather than stuck in the role of victim.

Injury and attack

> 'I dreamt that my school friends and I were being chased by wolves and when they caught us they would eat us.'
>
> Helen (5)

Helen's dream may have been triggered by the story of the Three Little Pigs, and it's always useful when trying to understand dreams to consider simple explanations rather than complex ones. Look for 'day residue', such as stories surfacing in dreams. If that doesn't connect, then consider what the dream animals symbolise and work through some of the techniques described earlier.

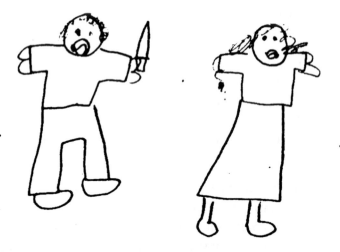

Girl Chased by Knifeman

Attack may come from any source: animals, aliens, or friends who 'shapeshift' into villains. 'Next to animals,' say American dream researchers and psychologists Calvin Hall and Vernon Nordby, 'the male stranger is the most frequent enemy of the dreamer and the one with whom the dreamer has the most serious transgressions.' Whatever or whoever the attacker, these dreams express vulnerability. They show how waking thoughts inspired by actual events, or news items and television dramas, trigger thoughts of 'What if that happened to me?' The dreams wrestle with issues of life and death and give us an opportunity to reassure children that we will protect them and to explain how unlikely such events are. Though attack and kidnap figure on news programmes, it is precisely because they are statistically rare that they get on the news. Yet attack is a common nightmare theme:

> 'I had a nightmare once about a man with a chainsaw and he chased me and my daddy round the town. He cut a lump out of my leg then I started screaming.'
>
> Claire (10)

> 'The most frightening dream I ever had was when I dreamt that a man with only half a face climbed up my drainpipe and in through my bedroom window. He picked up my sister's tights and strangled my sister and me.'
>
> Emma (9)

> 'In my dream I walked downstairs into the living room and this Alsatian dog flew at me – it had rabies or something – and it got me by my neck and just started shaking me all over the place as if I was a rag doll.'
>
> John (8)

In each of these dreams there is physical disfigurement in one form or another. There is also a lack of support: there is no champion to protect or rescue the dreamer. Children are at the mercy of the adult world and, for some, that mercy is not as kind as it might be. Some children feel isolated and vulnerable. Similarly, in Erin's dream there is no escape:

> 'The most frightening dream I ever had was that I was locked in a steel room then all of the walls and the ceiling started closing in.'
>
> Erin (10)

Erin had the dream when life was 'closing in' on her. There were problems in her family and she felt there was no escape from all the distress. Her dream symbolically represented her sense of being trapped. When children tell you about dreams like these, try to explore whether they feel vulnerable or under attack and use the techniques described at the end of this chapter to increase feelings of self-confidence.

Shapeshifting

As we grow up we learn that our heroes, our 'perfect' parents and others, are not always as wonderful as we want them to be. We learn that adults are complicated. They can be nice most of the time then transform into furious demons. In nightmares this transformation occurs in 'shapeshifting':

> 'I dream that men and women change into monsters and eat other people. They eat heads and arms and legs. I hate these bad dreams.'
>
> Paul (10)

> 'My most frightening dream was where my mum was in a hair-dressers and they poisoned her with shampoo. Then she came back and started to turn into an old fogey.'
>
> Sarah (9)

Julie had this dream when she was 7, and it includes both the transformation that occurs in shapeshifting and the sense of horror, as well as the pain of being disbelieved:

> 'The dream took place at my Nana's house. I walked into the large bedroom where my Nana sleeps and found my dad standing beside the bed dressed in trousers, shirt and tie, but he had a monster's head. His hair was on end, he had a greeny, grey disfigured face and he had large fangs dripping saliva. I was petrified. I just stood there shocked that my loving, caring dad had changed into an evil monster. I ran screaming into the living room where my mum was and told her what I saw. She laughed when we went into the bedroom because my dad was back to normal. When my mum started to laugh at me, for thinking my dad was a monster, I cried even more because I was annoyed because I really did see him and hurt because no one believed me.'

It helps children to recognise that we are each complex beings with positive and negative sides and that these 'shapeshifting' nightmares show us this in a dramatic way.

Post-traumatic nightmares

Linda (10) told me about a recurring nightmare that she has had since she was 5 years old: '…there is a man, a devil, taking me away. Then there are people coming after me trying to kill me.' Dreams she has now are also terrifying:

> 'There is me and a lady. I was crying. Catapulted into a lady's garden. Then a man is chasing me. He chopped me up.'

She sleepwalks, and was once nearly killed after walking out of the house late one night. The point at which the child first has the dream is often significant, as it is in Linda's case. When she was 5 she was sexually abused by a stranger who was subsequently imprisoned.

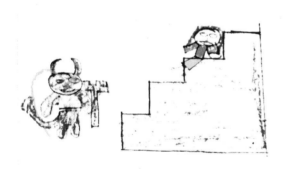

Girl and the Devil

Her dreams tell us that her very deep-seated fears have yet to be worked through. Professional help can be obtained through specialist agencies such as the school psychological service or the NSPCC, who have workers trained in counselling victims of sexual abuse.

Sexually abused children frequently develop post-traumatic stress disorder. British psychologist Neville King and his co-researchers described the experience of 'Sally' (10) whose abuse was recognised after she began to have severe sleep disturbance and recurrent nightmares, and behaved 'out of character'. Working with the nightmares was central to her treatment, as were teaching her relaxation techniques to relieve her anxiety and social skills training so that she was able to use assertive techniques to enhance her self-confidence.

Five-year-old Anthony lives in a family where there has been a history of abuse and neglect. His dreams reflect his distress and sense of being powerless. In his dreams skeletons chase him and his sister: 'The skeleton was going to eat me. I killed him but my sister was dead.' In fact his dreams were full of attacks, shootings, bombings and imagery that revealed an all-pervading sense of being under threat. If you look at his drawing of his dream 'Ghosts in my room'. He lies in his bed, a tiny figure without arms. He appears powerless, with no protection. The ghosts have no ears so cannot hear the cries that come from his open mouth. Symbolically no one has ears to listen.

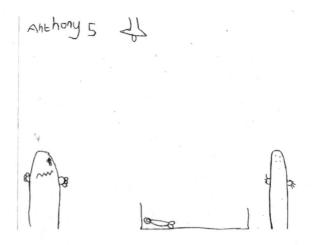

Ghosts in my Room

The kind of nightmare that Linda experiences is a special type of recurring, often literal, nightmare that follows overwhelmingly intense and unexpected outside events. They may continue for years but particularly at times when the dreamer is reminded of her past helplessness. Lenore Terr, a member of staff at the University of California School of Medicine, studied a group of 26 children who had been kidnapped from their school bus in Chowchilla, California, and then buried alive by their three abductors. They were held captive for about 27 hours. A year after their ordeal, and again four to five years later, the children, whose ages ranged from 5 to 14 years, still had nightmares which exactly repeated the trauma. Additionally, many of the group tended to walk, talk or scream in their sleep.

As time passed the Chowchilla children tended to elaborate the recurrent dreams of the kidnapping so that in some cases the original trauma became hidden underneath other material. However, such disguised nightmares still tell us that traumatic experiences deeply affect children's psyches and they need help to exorcise the pain. Other children who have had a psychologically overwhelming life event dream that they themselves die. Terr points out that personal-death dreams and recurrent nightmares often indicate that a traumatic event has taken place in the past, and these children allow themselves to die in their dreams because they no longer believe in personal invulnerability.

American psychologist Patricia Garfield, author of *Your Child's Dreams*, points out that films, TV and books may reactivate past traumas or stresses, making the individual attempt to face them once again. They may have old fears evoked with no help to deal with them; just reactivation, never clarification and completion.

Dealing with trauma

An intelligent and articulate girl from Dublin, Bridgit (8) has experienced a number of family tragedies. Her family friend, a woman 'who had been sad for a long time', hanged herself. Bridgit's family, hard pressed to make ends meet, moved to England, where she started at a new school. All these major life changes, life 'stressors', happened within four months. Her dreams reflect these traumas. Though her happiest dreams are about having nice clothes and being rich in a fairy-tale sort of way, the painful dreams are of a much darker hue:

'A nightmare about a man up in the sky with a dog with two heads on it. Mammy went out but she did not think the dog was alive. It was making her bleed. Mammy got a stick and broke it. The man up in the sky was happy. At the last bit, Mammy died…I dream of Maureen that died. She is shouting "I will get her", and has weapons to hurt me.'

Bridgit drew her dead friend lifting a sword and swinging a mace in the air ready to smash them down on the terrified child. In a way her friend has already dealt the blow, because the knowledge that her friend had taken her own life is a dreadful truth for Bridgit to contemplate. If adults on whom children rely act in such a way, how can children comprehend the world? Bridgit still seemed shell-shocked.

I was not able to work through this material with Bridgit. However, I was able to spend a little time with her talking about separation and loss, for she had lost her friend, her old school, her home and her country. There is much archetypal material in her dream. The two-headed dog is like Janus the 'January' god who sees the old and the new, the past and future. Dogs in ancient mythology were the companions of the dead on their 'night sea crossing' from the world of the living to the world of the dead. In symbolic terms the mace, a very unusual item to see in the dream of an 8-year-old, denotes a crushing blow or utter destruction, the annihilation of the assertive tendency in mankind, not merely victory over a foe. The intensity of this archetypal imagery tells us how grave an effect Bridgit's circumstances have had on her psyche. The indifference of the callous 'man-in-the-sky' god reveals a fear that there is not even a higher being who will give support.

Mangled by the media: 'Television with a nightmare on'

All over the world there are grave concerns about the influence of the media on children. Over 2500 studies have been conducted in America into the effects of television violence on the behaviour of viewers. The overall evidence was strong enough to persuade the Surgeon General of the USA to issue a report stating that television violence is dangerous to young people's health. By the time the average American child completes high school, she will have spent more time in front of the television set than in the classroom. By age 19 she will have seen 22,000 violent deaths on television.

There can be no doubt that television has a significant influence on the lives of children. In my research with over 800 children, I found that the extent and depth to which videos and television are invading the psyches of our children is phenomenal. Their dreams teem with images from the screen. The invasion of the mind-snatchers brings nightmares to our children.

At a special conference on media research and education held in Switzerland, media educator Miguel Reyes Torres asked a probing question: 'Imagine you come home from work and find a strange man talking to your 5- and 8-year-old children. Are you happy about this? The symposium gave Torres, and other concerned colleagues in Latin America, an opportunity to describe how their culture and values are being eroded by the invasion of foreign culture via the television set. For instance, more than 50 per cent of television programmes in Chile are imported from the USA, and it has been shown that parents there vastly underestimate the amount their children watch.

> 'These aliens came to earth. They pretended to be friendly, then they attacked, killing everybody except me, then one ate me. It started on my hand and slowly worked upwards and I couldn't stop it. Each alien had pointed ears and small beady eyes in a head too big for its body.'
>
> Donna (8)

In a survey carried out by head teachers, one nursery in five reported incidents of random violence. Neil Postman, professor of media ecology at New York University, pointed out that Americans are exposed to 800 commercials each week and that as consumers they are heavily influenced by this. The pervasive influence of TV, videos and films is all too evident in children's nightmares. When disturbing films are seen before sleep then there is a greater proportion of anxiety elements during REM sleep. One 10-year-old boy in all innocence grasped the confusion between the nightmare he dreamt and the vision on TV. When asked why he thought we dream, he replied: 'Because we watch television with a nightmare on.'

Very young children are greatly affected by material meant for adults, and even though they may at first object or show signs of distress, parents often ignore them. Kane (6) has recurring nightmares about:

> '…video dead…an electric saw. They sawed the monster's head off and then the monster got up and picked it up.'

This is a straight replay of the video watched with his parents. Now Kane's dream life is full of these overpowering images and he is afraid to go to sleep at night. His parents wonder what all the fuss is about and get angry with him. Kane is even more confused because he feels guilty that these films should upset him!

In my research children repeatedly articulated the sources of their nightmares. Martha (8): 'My dad gets a video out and I watch, then my nightmares are about the videos he gets out.' And Lisa (12) dreams 'I have nightmares after I have watched a horror film. I go to bed and dream that someone is going to rape and attack me and then throw me on to the railway line…'. Again and again children told me of nightmares that were directly related to something they had seen on TV or in films.

When I was working on my book *Women Dreaming*, I had a letter from a very worried mother:

> 'My son Lee is 6 years old and has for the past three months been having nightmares about a man with no face, but a lot of hair, who slashes at my son with his fingers and cuts him all over. My son then wakes up in tears, very, very upset and absolutely terri- fied. This man is very real to him.'

She was so worried that she contacted her son's doctor and teacher, who in turn spoke to her son, reassuring him that such a man was not real. Both professionals assured the mother that there was nothing wrong with her little boy but, she asked, 'What could possibly cause such dreams?' Had she asked some of her son's friends maybe they would have told her about Freddy, a very 'real' character known to many.

Freddy Krueger is the razor-gloved star of *A Nightmare on Elm Street*, which played to packed cinema audiences in the USA and Britain. The availability of videos for home viewing explains why such young children have seen, and been affected by, the film. Many children told me about him, they saw him attack, felt his gouging fingers and heard his words, and his scraping nails.

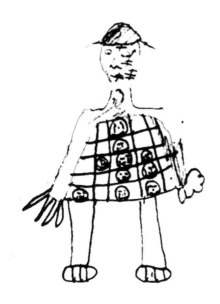

Freddy

What is it about Freddy that captured the psyches of the young? According to *Time* magazine, it is because Freddy symbolises what teenagers love to hate – their fathers! Part of the explanation lies in projection – that psychological phenomenon which allows us to put on to others, to 'project', feelings that we find too uncomfortable to own. So the viewer sees a highly dramatic acting out of his inner, maybe subconscious, violence, lust or cruelty. Young people project their feelings out on to others, and part of the process of growing up is learning to recognise and deal with those bits of ourselves that frighten or shame us.

Children expose themselves to frightening sensations, and by facing them learn to conquer the fear. That is a healthy thing to do. There is also an element of bravado – seeing horror movies proves that you can take it. However, it can become more problematic. Valerie Yule, a child psychologist working with disturbed children, found that as well as having a traumatic family history, most disturbed 7- and 8-year-olds had been constantly exposed to destruction and meaninglessness on television, without having the language to comprehend it. They were bombarded by violence but there was neither rhyme nor reason to it; violence for them was just an ordinary, accepted part of life.

Many authors from Edgar Allen Poe to Stephen King, and film makers such as Alfred Hitchcock and Ingmar Bergman, have frightened their audiences for years with their nightmare productions, which at times create a fantastic dream world. It is interesting to note that Poe, Hitchcock and Bergman all suffered severe trauma in childhood and the sense of being overwhelmed and powerless in the face of trauma is transmitted in their imagery. As psychiatrist Christian Guilleminault says: 'The audience accepts the helpless panic and goes to bed to dream its bad dreams. Horror is contagious. It can be experienced by those who never themselves were directly horrified.' Children need not see the offending films themselves; others may well tell them, spread the contagion of fear, and as if by proxy the dreams occur, as in the case of Lee, the 6-year-old who had nightmares about Freddy. If your child has nightmares and you don't watch this type of video at home, find out if he watches them at sleepovers.

Heavy viewers of television violence believe that the level of violence in the world is much higher than given by actual statistics. Research from the USA, Israel, Finland, Poland and Australia shows how at certain times during a child's development, extensive exposure to television violence promotes aggressive behaviour in the child. American psychologists Rowell Huesmann and Leonard Eron gathered data over 22 years, following 8-year-olds through to age 30. They discovered that the critical age range was 6 to 11; chillingly they concluded: '... aggressive habits that are established during this time are resistant to extinction and often persist into adulthood... More aggressive children watch more violence and that viewing seems to engender more aggression.' This applies especially to those boys who have poorer academic skills. They watch TV violence more regularly, behave more aggressively, and believe that the violent programmes they watch depict life as it truly is.

Huesmann and Eron also found that childhood aggression learnt from violent TV shows interferes with later intellectual development and may actually diminish adult cognitive achievement. So not only do they trigger nightmares, they hinder later progress. Aggression interferes with academic success because it causes difficulties with peers and teachers alike, further alienating the young person who thus becomes more isolated and in turn watches more TV. A vicious circle can develop in which TV becomes the fix and the viewer becomes the addict. This reinforces the aggression, and new aggressive schemes or codes are learnt and stored. For boys the effect was exacerbated by the degree to which the boy identified with TV characters.

Night terrors

Night terrors, also known as *pavor nocturnus*, are usually seen in early childhood and rarely continue beyond puberty, which may give some consolation to parents whose children suffer from them. They are caused by a dysfunction as the brain moves from one level of sleep to another. Night terrors are different from nightmares; with night terrors you may find yourself woken by a screaming, disoriented child, who is the very picture of abject terror. Although you try to reason with your wide-eyed child he may not recognise you, or he may be completely incoherent.

Other signs of night terrors are heavy breathing, distorted facial features, perspiration and moving around as if to escape whatever it is that is so terrifying. Such an episode may last 10 or 15 minutes, after which time the child settles back to sleep. Usually he has completely forgotten the incident in the morning and will be surprised if told about it. However, this may not always be the case, as I have spoken to both adults and children who recall their night terrors.

Although only about 3 per cent of children experience night terrors, this sleep disorder does give cause for concern. Research by Bryan Lask, a consultant psychiatrist at Great Ormond Street Hospital in London, looks particularly promising. He asked parents to observe exactly when their child had night terrors. On the nights following the five observation sessions the parents woke the child 10 to 15 minutes before the expected terror was due. After five minutes the child was allowed to go back to sleep. This waking routine was to be stopped when the terrors ceased. Over a year after this intervention took place, there were no relapses: the 19 children who took part remained night-terror free.

Strategies to banish nightmares

As 9-year-old Uzma said, 'nightmares hurt your feelings'. So, we need to find ways to prevent such hurt feelings. These techniques will help you to help children understand their nightmares. What can you do?

- *Listen* – First and foremost listen to the child. Show you value their dreams, their ideas and their feelings by taking time to hear what they have to say.

- *Draw the dream* – Children enjoy drawing their dreams. Look at the picture together. Let the child give it a title. Let her explain what is happening. Ask her what would make the nightmare feel less scary. Put in a 'helper' if the child thinks that would help or cut out the offending monster.

- *Act out the dream* – Create a play to re-enact the dream. Let the child play the bad characters as well as the others. Ask 'How does it feel to be the monster?' The child may identify parts of herself or enjoy the feeling of power. Perhaps there are times in the child's life when she feels angry, wants to chase someone, etc. Link it to waking life if appropriate.

- *Interview the monster* – Let the child pretend she is a newspaper reporter or television interviewer. Ask her to put a few questions to the monster. You, of course will be her guard and protect her. If the child finds that too frightening, she can imagine the monster is in gaol, behind bars, so she can safely speak to him. Ask questions such as 'Why were you chasing Jane?', 'What did you want from Jane?', etc. Then the child pretends to be the monster and answers. Often the monster says 'I only wanted to talk to her because I'm lonely' or 'Jane was horrible to me and I wanted to get my own back.' Then explore waking life connections.

- *Confront the monster* – Imagine the monster is there in front of both you and the child. Ask her what she wants to say to him and both of you say it. For instance, 'Get out of my dreams and don't come back!' Don't just say it, YELL IT!

- *Reinforce your dream palace* – The 'dream palace' referred to here is the child's bedroom! Throughout history we have used amulets and talismans to protect ourselves. In Ancient Egypt, the midget god Bes had the job of protecting the household from nightmares. With his smiling face and jolly temperament he drove out the terrors. His likeness was carved into bedheads and headrests. Children could make their own happy nightmare figures to act as protectors.

- *Make a dream catcher* – A 'dream catcher' is a Native American introduction. A ring or hoop is decorated with thread and a 'web' is woven across the centre, and feathers, beads and other ornamentation attached. It is said that the dream catcher keeps hold of good dreams while allowing the bad ones to disappear. When you have made the dream catcher you can then hang it at the child's bedroom window.

Here's another technique to deal with nightmares. I came across it in Norwegian child psychotherapist Torben Marner's book *Letters to Children in Family Therapy*. In one of his letters to a little girl he had worked with he described how nightmares are a little stupid – nightmares think they are bringing interesting, exciting dreams. Also, nightmares are very curious so it is easy to outwit them. He suggests that the child gets hold of a box with a keyhole: when the nightmare comes it will see the box, and instead of bothering the child it will slip into the box. But because it is stupid, the nightmare won't be able to find its way out again! Then, Marner suggests, every so often the child goes with his parents into the countryside to let the nightmares out of the box.

This technique works well because it gives the child control and it involves the parents as helpful partners. If you are working with a group of children you could make individual 'nightmare boxes' out of cardboard boxes, cut out keyholes and decorate them. It's fun to stick on glitter, sequins, gold and silver twine, and so on, to 'attract' the curious nightmares. Also, the addition of luminous stars would shine out for the child in a dark bedroom, which would reassure and comfort her.

And finally, a couple of ideas from children themselves:

> 'When I was young I always used to 'nightmare' about things like skeletons or baddies, usually after watching a film. Now, I have taught myself to – before I go to sleep – think of nice things. My

favourite one is holidays: villas in the Algarve, sun-blistered beaches in Spain, white waters in Canada…'

Matt (12)

'I realised in childhood when I decided whilst awake to face the frightening thing in the dream and then I did it in the dream, the fear dispelled.'

Noel (15)

'When I have scary dreams about ghosts and monsters. I tell my mum and now I pray.'

Kerry-Anne (9)

'Put a notice on the door saying: No Bad Dreams, Only Friendly Monsters and Jolly Giants.'

Zara (10)

If after trying to reassure your child you find he is still having night terrors or sleep problems over several weeks and continues to be distressed, then do seek the advice of your doctor. Severe problems can be treated and you may well need to find support for yourself as well as your child.

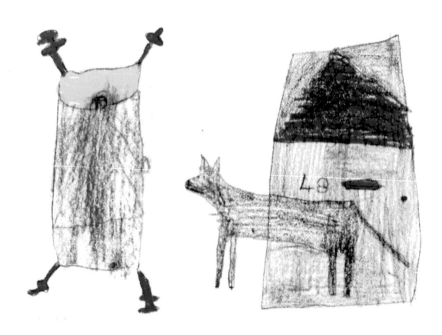

The Dog Came in When I Was in Bed

Chapter Seven

Creative Dreaming

Dreams, creative expression and the soul are inseparable.
Jill Mellick, *The Natural Artistry of Dreams*

A dream is a gift. It comes to us unbidden and can bring with it freedom to fly, to swim under water, to meet speaking animals and to experience that which we have not even imagined. For children, as for adults, this enhances creativity and lets the spirit sing.

When we work with dreams we travel with an open mind. Each dream is unique and as we celebrate that we open up to creative potential. In dreams we can occupy two time frames: we can be our current age yet have the body of a younger child; we can be a different sex; we can shapeshift to exotic creatures; and we can converse with those who have died. In developing creativity in children, all of these can be used in art forms: story telling, myth making, drawing, painting and drama. The spirit of inquiry and curiosity are the keys to working with dreams creatively. Research in education has shown that creativity can be taught; it is not merely an innate talent or lucky genes, and for all our futures we need children whose creativity has been nurtured.

Children and creativity

Most children have what Jungian analyst Marie-Louise von Franz calls 'no unconscious doubt'. They don't have that censorious barrier between impulse and expression. A young child will draw a face on the wallpaper of his bedroom because that seems a perfectly OK place to do it. She draws her friend with blue hair riding on a horse that flies through the skies and sees no problem with that. Her imagination soars and she thrives on its expression. All too soon, killjoys come along and say 'Horses can't fly' or 'Hair isn't that colour'. We need to be tender with the glorious creative spontaneity our children express and accept that they enjoy the process and are not focused on the outcome. We need to trust the process.

Encourage children to dream and learn from their dreams and to:

- explore
- play with
- respect
- be with the dream
- day-dream about
- take flight with
- connect
- immerse in
- doodle with
- experience
- develop a dream language
- build their own symbol lists
- create a zoo of dream creatures
- create a gallery of dream characters
- paint dreamscapes
- learn to love the puzzle
- experiment
- make a mandala

- sculpt the dream settings
- make masks to ward off nightmare monsters
- participate in dream plays
- share ideas
- let dreams be launching pads
- let dreams be resting places
- accept the mystery of dreams
- respect the boundless possibility of our dream world
- enjoy.

Writing about dreams

Literary inspiration

Throughout history writers have found a rich vein of material in their dreams. Poet and diarist Maya Angelou and horror writer Clive Barker told American writer Naomi Epel about the importance of dreams as inspiration for their work. She wrote a book called *Writers Dreaming* that includes a wealth of material for anyone who wants to use dreams as a part of the creative process.

Many writers have taken images or motifs from dreams, including Isabel Allende and W.B. Yeats. Graham Greene at the age of 8 had a vivid dream of a disastrous shipwreck; he later discovered that the *Titanic* went down that night. In his book *A Sort of Life* he tells how important his dreams have been to him, including many that were either telepathic or precognitive, especially concerning disasters and death.

Robert Louis Stevenson was racking his brains for a plot to show how man can be transformed when he had a dream: 'I dreamed a scene at the window, and a scene afterwards split into two, in which Hyde, pursued for some crime, took the powder and underwent the change in the presence of his pursuers.' Thus, the classic *Dr Jekyll and Mr Hyde* was conceived. Another classic was born when Mary Shelley dreamt of the 'hideous phantasm' which was to enter the public world in the shape of her novel *Frankenstein*.

Creative dream writing

These are ways you can build on the energy of dreams using words:

- Write the dream in circles or start at the edges of the paper going into the centre as you write it down.

- Use different coloured pens or pencils for each dream section.

- Use the main dream image as a template – a dream of a house could be written with certain words in the roof, other parts in the window spaces, yet more in the door, and so on.

- Write about the dream diagonally across the page.

- Let the dream wander over the page.

- Write the dream on different pieces of paper then assemble them (In the right order? Randomly?) What do you come up with?

- Make a book. Write each section of the dream on a separate sheet. Illustrate it. Add drawings, magazine cut-outs and postcards and assemble into a book. Give it a title.

- Make a personal or group 'dream library'.

- The most important words can be written LARGE and LOUD.

- Choose three words from the dream and grow them.

  > 'I am in a maze of rocks and there's a big hole below me and someone is chasing me.'
  >
  > Noel (10)

  - *maze* – hard to find your way out, labyrinth, amazing
  - *rocks* – beach, countryside, climbing, getting over them
  - *hole* – falling, Alice in Wonderland, dark place, going to the earth's centre.

  Then make a story or poem using these words. It's another way of exploring and honouring the dream.

- What happens when you take out a character or object from the dream? How does it change? Write a story about where that character goes.

Dream inventions

Some of the most significant inventions have arisen from dreams, including Einstein's theory of relativity He had a dream when he was a boy in which he was tobogganing down a hill. He saw the way the light seemed to bend and was so fascinated by it that he made it his life's work to discover what made light bend.

The Marquis de Saint-Denys living in the 19th century was sure that dreams create new inventions. He described one dream, about a transparent cat, which will interest many children:

> I see the animal gradually lose its initial appearance, becoming luminous, translucent, diaphanous and finally like glass itself... It swims, stretches out and then catches a mouse, as transparent as itself, which I hadn't noticed before; and as a result of the curious transformation of the two creatures, I see the remains of the unfortunate rodent descending into the stomach of its ferocious enemy. (quoted in van der Castle 1994, p.16)

He could never see anything like that in waking life, he said; his dream had invented it.

Without dreams the modern-day sewing machine may not have been invented when it was. Elias Howe wrestled with the design of a needle that would operate successfully. Frustrated and about to give up he went to bed with the problem on his mind. He dreamt that he was being chased by men who threw spears at him; at the end of each spear was a hole. He knew then he had to put the hole at the pointed end of his sewing machine needle, and so modern machining, which transformed the clothing industry, was invented.

> 'When we fall asleep all our imagination mixes with the things our brains remember.'
>
> Trixie (9)

Art

Dreams have inspired people to create great works of art since the time of the cave dwellers. Many painters have seen images in their dreams which were then transposed to canvas or in sculpture. Arthur Rackham, a great

British illustrator and painter whose work enhanced children's books, used inspirational dreams as the source of much of his work. William Blake, English poet, artist and visionary, was profoundly influenced by his dreams. Many of the titles of his paintings and engravings reflect this, such as 'Queen Catherine's Dream', 'Oh, How I Dreamt of Things Impossible' and the pencil portrait 'The Man Who Taught Blake Painting In His Dreams'. Blake also described how his dead brother came to him in a dream to teach him an extraordinary engraving technique which allowed him to produce the luminous works which ensured his lasting fame. The Surrealist group of artists deliberately tried to recreate the dream state by juxtaposing unusual objects that would not normally be put together. A good example of this is René Magritte's painting 'Golconde', in which bowler-hatted men drop from the sky instead of raindrops. Others such as Salvador Dali, Max Ernst and Odilon Redon explored the mysterious world of dreams in their creations.

Creative art work

Use the dream as a basis for collage work. Cut shapes out to represent different parts of the dream, make head shapes with smiles or frowns to represent feelings, symbolically depict power by hats, for example a crown, mortar board, baseball cap or a Sherlock Holmes-type hat for the investigator. Masks can be used in the same way.

Here is a sample dream and some ways to develop it.

> 'In my dream I went to a party and ended up being chased by a wolf only I could see.'
>
> Anna (10)

Get some big, thick crayons or paints, fat paint brushes and a large sheet of paper.

- Depict the wolf using the *non-dominant* hand. This frees the child up to make a less than perfect representation. It also produces a raw energy which really sets the creative process alive.

- Get a plastic tray and half fill it with sand. Let the child draw the wolf 'only she could see' and then let her choose to let others see it or to wipe it away without anyone seeing it.

- Use a glue stick to draw the wolf on paper or card then sprinkle on sand or glitter or lentils so the image emerges.

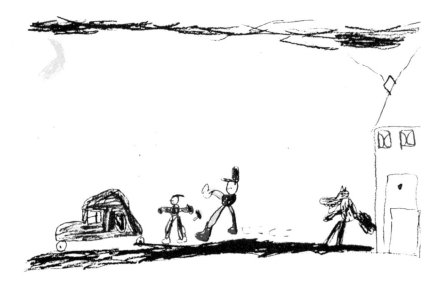

Chased by Wolf

These techniques are part of the process of honouring the idea of visibility. They allow an image to arise, to come from the invisible and let the child explore the sense of being seen and not being visible which is part of her dream experience.

Some other things to explore when dream animals appear:

- Habitat – where does it usually live?

- Tamed or wild?

- What does it eat? How does it get its food?

- What kind of fur or skin does it have?

- Solitary or gregarious?

- How does it travel?

- How long does it live?
- Strengths and weaknesses?
- How does it get along with other animals?
- Have you ever seen this animal? In the flesh or on TV?
- Can you think of any phrases that describe this animal?

Honour the dream:

- Collect pictures of the animal and make a collage.
- Work with a group to brainstorm ideas, feelings and connections others make to the dream animal.
- Can you make any mythological or fairy-story connections?
- Explore the lifespan of the animal. Make a diagram.

This way of amplifying or enriching the dream images develops the child's confidence in his own creativity. Finally, write a story for other children about the dream animal including some of the elements that have come from thinking about the dream.

> 'I was in bed and there was a spider in the corner of the bedroom and it grew and grew and actually tried to eat me up.'
>
> Ruth (8)

Fairy-stories

Dreams make wonderful ingredients for the development of fairy-stories which in turn foster the child's imagination, language skills and all-round creativity. Some dreams already have a very mythical dimension, which we see in this one that 12-year-old Vanessa had:

> 'I was in another land with waterfalls and long green grass and a forest and a palace made of gold. A young servant marries a prince in the palace. Every night they sit by a river in the full of the moon and I am the owl watching from a tree.'

Already a great outline for a fairy-tale. In more mundane dreams, however, where such creativity is not so immediately apparent, there are some basic techniques which help in the writing process which you will see in the box

'Make your own dream fairy-tales'. Let's see how it works with Daksha's dream.

> 'I dreamt that all the fishes took over the people. The fishes had swords and were killing us, then I woke up.'
>
> Daksha (12)

Make your own dream fairy-tales

- Begin with 'Once upon a time'.
- Set your story in the past and in a place far away.
- Give the characters significant names that begin with capitals.
- Build things up or shrink them – exaggerate.
- Give extra details about clothes, places and people.
- Let magical things happen – animals can talk, people can fly.
- Provide helpers – guides, angels, power animals and potions.
- Add dialogue.
- Invent things and include them to add excitement.
- Let your imagination run riot; anything can happen.
- Give it an enticing title.
- Add a moral. What has your chief character discovered that is important?

Here is a development of the story using some of the techniques listed.

The Heavenly Dolphins

Once upon a time, in a land far beyond the mountains, lived Queen Ahskad, who was good and kind. The Heavenly Palace where she lived with King Phindol was built of white marble and surrounded by glorious palm trees, white sand and a calm, turquoise sea. Everyone who worked in the Heavenly Palace was richly paid and all the people of the land were happy. They ate ripe fruit, swam in the sea, lounged about in the sun and had the best life it was possible to imagine.

One day the Queen woke up and told her husband of a strange dream she had:

'It was stormy and gigantic waves rushed towards the beach,' she said in a shaking voice. 'It was so terrible that I forced myself awake.'

The King counselled her to think no more of the dream and called for breakfast to be served in the beautiful bedroom overlooking the turquoise sea. As they sat eating fresh mangoes, there was a huge commotion. Poseidon, their enormous dog jumped from his couch and dashed on to the balcony. His barks deafened their ears before he took up the fierce pose of a guard dog. Servants ran in to see if their beloved Queen and King were under attack, and once they saw the dog they waited for his warning.

'Look! See the glinting and flashing in the water?' gasped the Queen.

King Phindol pointed out to the sea. 'I can see giant swords and scimitars cutting the sky.'

The sea was no longer turquoise. It was a mass of swirling orange waves topped with black crests. Suddenly, the dog's growling message filled the ominous silence as all the people in the Heavenly Palace turned their gaze from the terrifying tidal wave that was threatening their perfect world. The wisest dog in their land spoke.

'Fish fever, sword danger. King Phindol, you must reclaim your powers for enemies draw near.'

The fairy-tale could go many ways from here, but you get the picture! Notice how Daksha has become the central character Ahskad, which is an anagram of her name. The King's name is an anagram for dolphin, and obviously he will have the same characteristics of intelligence, knowledge of the seas, and so on, that are needed to bring the story to a positive ending. The magic dog knows this, and we can assume all will be well in the end. You could use this beginning as a way of demonstrating how we can use dreams as the basis for fairy-stories and perhaps think about or write out the rest of the tale. (If you do, I'd love to see the results – contact details are on the final page.)

Myths

Myths and legends are stories handed down from generation to generation and were believed to be true. Myths are relevant to dreams and creativity since they deal with the same themes. Many ancient myths and legends involve puzzles and riddles which the hero/heroine has to solve. Such tests put an awesome burden on the puzzler and a high price on failure. We can see this in Jodie's dream:

> 'I dream about being in the devil's house doing puzzles to keep my mum alive and I always try to change the dream into something nice because it is horrible.'

Jodie (12), who lives in a small village in Ireland, has a number of dreams that involve her taking responsibility for her mother in some way. She also has a recurring dream that her mother falls off a bridge, and she has to dive in the river to save her. At a deep, unconscious level she seems to be afraid that her mother is at risk in some way, and she is prompted constantly to seek assurances that her mother is all right.

If you would like further ideas on how to use writing with dreams I recommend Jill Mellick's wonderful book *The Natural Artistry of Dreams*.

Creating success – Rehearsal dreams

Sports are a regular feature of children's dreams. For Jillian (7), her happiest dream was one in which she was swimming club champion in her age group. She was thrilled with the dream, which boosted her confidence, and she said, 'It came true.' John (10) was not such a good swimmer but a dream helped him too:

> 'When I started to learn to swim, I knew the stroke but did it much too fast and kept sinking. I was desperate to learn. One night I dreamed I was swimming doing the stroke slowly and enjoying it. Next day I got in the water and swam right across the pool.'

Alison (10) dreamt that she won a cup on her pony Breeze. She said, 'I felt really excited and when I woke up it felt like it was really true.' This kind of dream helps a child feel more self-assured, as if they have rehearsed a challenge and come through successfully. Richard told me that we dream because 'if we don't do well in real life we have a second chance'.

Such dreams are not confined to sporting events:

'When my mum and dad got divorced I tried to get them together again and in my dreams I thought about how to go about it.'

Fiona (10)

Jennifer (13) explained how her dreams helped:

'In my dream I imagined that I was going to improve my looks. So in my dream I made my hair really lovely and that's what I did the next day after my dream... I have psoriasis and one night I dreamt of myself really working hard at putting my treatment on. So when I woke up I got the urge to always keep on putting on the cream, day and night.'

Using dreams to help prepare for future events is not new. Napoleon used his dreams to help him prepare for battles. On waking he would write down his dreams and test the strategies using toy soldiers to plot his campaigns. The dreams provided the key, which he then translated into waking action.

Next, we turn to dreams that have a special part to play in children's health.

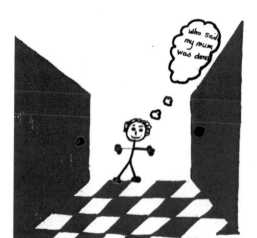

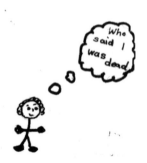

Who Said my Mum was Dead?

Chapter Eight

The Impact of Illness and Disability

My most frightening dream was when I was ill and I thought I
was never going to get better.

Vikki (9)

Our dreams can help us with our physical, emotional and spiritual health,
as people have known for thousands of years. As early as 3000 BC we have
written records of dreams that were used in both the diagnosis of illness
and its treatment. In Ancient Greece and Egypt, where the practice of
dream incubation took place, people would sleep in special temples in
deliberate attempts to induce inspirational, divine and healing dreams.
Hippocrates, the father of modern medicine, Aristotle and Plato all
believed that dreams revealed unseen workings of body and soul.

It was not only diagnosis and prognosis of illness that concerned the
early Greeks, but healing as well. There were 420 Asklepian temples at one
time scattered throughout Greece, and when a person was ill she would go
to such a temple, perform certain rites, sleep in a sanctified chamber and
wait for a healing dream. They believed that Asklepios, the god of healing,
would appear in the dream and effect a cure. Nowadays such temples have
fallen into ruins, but the power of dreams in relation to illness has not.
Changes in the body are registered in the unconscious before our waking
brains have noticed them and these subliminal changes are found in the
dreams of family, friends or doctor before the 'patient' has an inkling of

any change. Dreams may warn of impending illness, or help the dreamer to face emotions repressed during waking hours.

Dreams that warn of illness are known as 'prodomic' dreams, from the Greek meaning 'to run before'. Toni (12) described how, two days before she is sick, she has warning dreams. Robert C. Smith, of the University of Rochester Medical Centre in New York, in his research with adult hospital patients with life-threatening conditions, found that dreams do react to biologic functioning. Putting it very simply, he found that patients whose illnesses became fatal had significantly different dreams: men had more references to death, while women had more themes of separation in their dreams. However, this does not mean that a dream of death signifies a fatal illness!

> 'The night before my birthday I dreamt of a hospital and there was someone I knew in the bed. In the morning we went to school and when I got home my neighbours told me that Zita had broken her arm and is in hospital. I had to go to the hospital to get my present.'
>
> Matthew (9)

Matthew was puzzled about the fact that the dream came before Zita's accident. Whether there was a subliminal awareness that she was playing a dangerous game that might lead to a accident I'm not sure, but it is worth noting that many children do describe what appear to be precognitive dreams. You can learn more about this in Chapter 10.

Childhood ailments

When children have high temperatures and feverish symptoms, intensely vivid dreams are often recalled, often involving some form of distortion:

> 'When I am ill I dream about faces, people with swollen heads and small faces, floating about in my mind. The faces are of people I know like my mum and dad and my family. In the background, large and small shapes are also floating around. When I wake up I am sweating.'
>
> Anastasia (12)

Fire themes also appear when children have high temperatures:

'I dream that my body is being burned and I am still alive and trying to get out. Then I wake up.'

Betsy (11)

'Sometimes when I'm ill I dream about a huge bonfire and a clock. I fly into the clock and I can't breathe.'

Duncan (9)

The physical symptoms are translated into fiery images which simultaneously depict the child's anxiety.

Chicken pox

Chicken pox is a nasty childhood disease, and one which all of my three children had. My 5-year-old daughter was very frightened when she saw the 'pox' popping up and thought they would never go away! It took much reassurance to persuade her that she would not be covered in the painful blisters for ever. Charlotte (7) had her most frightening dream when she came down with chicken pox, and it seems to sum up the physical aspect of the illness. She said she was being chased by a giant:

'In my dream, every time I hit an island, it went bump! And then I hit another island and it went bump!'

This went on all night and when she woke she was covered in her 'bumps'.

Migraine

The psychologist Meredith Sabini quotes research into illnesses as diverse as arthritis, cancer, migraine and multiple sclerosis, in which dreams have aided understanding of the development of the illness and the patient's attitude to it. Migraine may start in childhood and dreams often warn of impending attacks. Pre-migraine dreams frequently involve anger, misfortune, fear and aggression as described in the research by American counsellors Gail Heather-Greener and her colleagues. If you regularly listen to your children's dreams you may find a pattern in which pre-migraine dreams feature. You can then see if you can avoid the attack, or take steps to minimise its effect.

Asthma

Fran was 5 when this dream first entered her life:

> 'These gloves appeared from nowhere and they kept coming in
> funny magician type moves. At first I thought it was fun watching
> them but then they would come close and start choking me. Then
> they would float back in the air again and start choking me again.'

The dream has stayed with her for seven years and came when she had her
first asthma attack. It recurs whenever she is asthmatic and symbolically
represents the sensations of being unable to breathe that she feels at these
times.

> 'When I am ill I usually have boxed-in sort of dreams where I feel
> trapped and short of air.'
>
> Katie (10)

Childhood asthma attacks often occur during the night, and studies by
Harold Levitan have shown that upsetting dreams play a part in their
onset. If the child has had a stressful, conflict-ridden day, then she is likely
to have disturbing dreams that may provoke an asthmatic attack. Clearly,
physical factors are important triggers too, but psychological factors are
known to be crucial: particularly relevant is the relationship with parents.
Twice as many boys suffer from asthma as girls, and this seems linked to
their feelings of aggression and deep conflicts: the active expression of
aggression in dreams seems to contribute to the production of asthma
attacks.

If you can bring these feelings into the light of day and deal with them
openly, difficult as this can be, you will help your child avoid night-time
asthma attacks. Children need help to accept that human beings come with
the full range of emotions from love to anger, from sorrow to joy. Part of
the maturation process involves learning how to unpack them and experience them positively.

Images in illness

Abstract forms of colour and shape are very common in the dreams of sick
children. They dream of lots of colours 'spinning round like a whirlwind'.

For some, 'writing appears on the bedroom wallpaper' or giant letters of the alphabet chase them. Andrew (11) combines these elements in his dreams during illness: 'I dream of patterns like white paper with red, purple, green and other colour blotches.' Things become less clear, unfocused, indicating perhaps changes in our ability to differentiate clearly objects and ideas when we are ill.

Ingrid (11) had a recurring dream during illness, which started when she was much younger. It too involves swirling round very fast in darkness, but:

> 'all of a sudden it would go so bright that I couldn't see. I would be going towards a brightly coloured triangle and just as I'm about to hit it, I wake up.'

Sometimes the colours are linked to a threat of some kind, as Alison (12) knows. This was the earliest dream she could remember and it still recurs when she is ill.

> 'My Mr Men curtain design changing into coloured blobs, coming out at me. In the background there was a man laughing and always there was a creamy white sheet of BIG paper that got blackened and dirtied which upset me.'

Kevin (11) has a recurring dream that small rocks, then larger rocks, come rolling down a hill to the bottom, where he is tied up. Before they hit him he wakes up. This type of dream shows how powerless we feel at the onset of illness. Kevin cannot prevent the onslaught, just as when we are 'run down' we do not have the strength to combat infection. Another kind of invasiveness is depicted in the dream of David (9) where he is 'in a land with green dust everywhere and green swampy slime dripping down from the trees'.

Fear of death

> 'When I am ill I dream that I will die.'
>
> Cathy (10)

Derry (11) made a heartfelt plea for understanding and support when he knew I was writing this book. He asked me to tell parents that 'when a child is ill he has very bad nightmares'. Derry only has nightmares when he is ill. He dreams that he dies, which is a common feature of children's dreams when they are unwell. Adults easily overlook the impact of illness on children; we take it for granted that they will recover. But for children the new experience is unknown and frightening.

> 'I dream about my friends being very ill and even dying. And they make me feel as if they are true and I sometimes wake up to find myself crying.'
>
> Valerie (10)

> 'When I was ill with my throat I dreamt that I was going to swallow my tonsils and choke on them. Then I dreamt I was going to die because I had nothing to drink and I was choking. My face went blue and I died.'
>
> Kelly (11)

Perhaps just a simple explanation of how infections cause swellings would help Kelly. She would understand that although she feels as if she is choking, she can still breathe because other airways are open for her and that her tonsils cannot become detached as they do in the dream. Plain facts help because children may be ignorant about how their bodies work.

Dreaming of death during illness is not at all uncommon for children, yet such fears are so easily overlooked. Consultant paediatrician, Simon Yudkin, said in his *Lancet* article 'Children and death': 'Some children who are ill are afraid of dying. They should be given the opportunity to show their fears and talk about what death means to them so that the origin of their worries can be made clear and so they can be reassured.'

The range of 'death' dreams during illness is often morbid: Xanthe (13) dreams that she will die 'without saying goodbye'; Gareth (12) dreams of his coffin and funeral; while Tabitha (12) dreams that she bequeaths all her money to her parents. She explained that when she is ill she always thinks about dying, so 'because I have it on my mind during the day, I dream about it at night'.

These dreams of death during illness would seem to have a very negative effect, but for Sally (13) this is not the case, for her dream of dying when ill 'is a funny sort of dream, yet I never die in it. I wake up upset and it gives me a will to get better'. Her dream encourages her to fight her illness and we know that fighting spirit is crucial for recovery to full health.

Love and medicine

Katy (12) has dreamt when ill that she is dying and that the only cure is a kiss from her mother. Remember the power of kisses to make hurts better? For Katy it appears there is still a great deal of investment in the power of her mother to heal her. Other children have other 'dream cures'.

Claire (11) has a lot dreams about fairies who grant wishes. When she had flu she dreamt that a fairy came through her window and threw magic dust over her. She said: 'When I woke up in the morning I was completely cured.' Bethany (7) dreamt of going to heaven and speaking to her grandad, which made her feel better straight away. Support from those whom they love is very important to children, especially sick children. And it does not matter if the person the child dreams of is dead, what is important is to recognise that the love of that person has been internalised by the child, and she carries it around inside like a charm to combat misfortune. The love we give children is the most powerful medicine available to each of us.

Chris (11) is certain that his dreams are therapeutic:

> 'I dream of getting better and the dream normally has something to do with it. For example, when I broke my arm I imagined being a weight-lifter.'

This dream seemed to strengthen his arm and he was optimistic about his dream-assisted recovery. 'Dream rehearsal' is a very useful technique to use with children. It is empowering and goes along with the holistic approach to health that recognises that mind and body work together to combat illness. Similarly Germaine (9) always has warrior dreams, which leave her feeling more confident that she will fight off her attacking illness.

Many children's dreams reveal a distrust of doctors and their remedies; they dream that the doctor or the prescribed medicine will kill them. Where a child tells you about this sort of dream, obviously you need to explain what the medicine will do and offer reassurance.

Feeling alone

Illness separates us from others, not just in the event of quarantine, but just because we cannot do ordinary things, it debilitates us. Children find this quite overpowering at times, partly because, with young children in particular, their sense of time is not developed and the duration of the illness seems like eternity. Children need daily reassurance and progress reports. I think Shaista (11) catches the mood of being 'kidnapped' by illness very well:

> 'When I am ill I dream about scary things like catching a very bad disease. Once I dreamed that I had to swap teeth with a man who kidnapped me. The teeth kept falling out so I had to use Superglue to stick them in.'

She is being forced to give up her own 'teeth', symbolically used to denote strength, and use another person's teeth. Is this 'other' person the doctor? Whatever or whoever it is, she needs additional help in order to retain her 'bite'. However, the dream has an optimistic atmosphere as she assertively finds a solution; she literally sticks with it!

Hospitals

> 'I was in hospital with fluid on my knee and they had to take it out so they brought me to the operating theatre and gave me an anaesthetic to go to sleep. When I was asleep I dreamt they were going to cut off my leg with a chainsaw.'
>
> Gemma (11)

Some children are very anxious when they go to hospital. Separated from people they trust and love and thrust into an alien environment, they become frightened that they will be physically hurt or changed. This is not a new finding. In 1945 Dr David Levy was the first child psychiatrist to recognise the significance of recurrent nightmares following operations. He compared the effects of the 'surgical field' to the battlefield, both of which may cause severe trauma expressed in nightmares.

Psychologist Lindy Burton describes the recurring nightmare of a 19-year-old student, which she traced to an experience at 3 years of age. The girl believed that the emergency operation for appendicitis had maimed her: 'Like so many other small children subjected to unexplained and often frightening illness and treatment procedures, she had evolved a fantasy in which her surgery had subtly but permanently damaged her.'

Children have all sorts of fears about surgery: that the anaesthetic will kill them or that the nurses want to harm them, administering, as they have to, unpleasant treatments. Later, lingering fears may be expressed directly in words, or more obliquely in behaviour. We can see this when children are so agitated that they cannot be still, when they have angry outbursts or look scared or withdraw into isolated shells, cutting themselves off from others. Similarly, a child who suddenly starts wetting or soiling the bed when she is normally dry, is communicating her distress by the change in behaviour. Dreams reflect these feelings too.

These fight (angry outbursts) or flight (withdrawal) behaviours are fear responses that can alert us to the child's distress. A child may feel a great sense of helplessness in illness, as if she has no control over her body or her life. It is a very frightening sensation and, if left unaided, it can lead to hopelessness, which further works against regaining health. Studies of the immune system described by the English biologist, Dr Paul Martin in *The Sickening Mind* show that the psychological willingness to combat disease brings about a high degree of successful rejection of illness, while passive acceptance is much less favourable in terms of recovery. Helping our children to fight illness positively is a health-giving strategy that benefits them throughout their lives.

Many parents who are reading this will have felt this anger from their children who have had to receive hospital treatment. It is often directed at mothers because young children expect her to be all-powerful and able to protect them from everything. In their unconscious disappointment, they hit out at the person to whom they are closest. Mother failed because she did not stop the pain or the operation, and left the child with strangers.

In their book *Emotional Care of Hospitalized Children* Madeline Petrillo and Sirgay Sanger discuss the case of 5-year-old Ruth. Ruth developed nightmares after cardiac surgery in America. When she returned from intensive care 48 hours after her operation, she refused to sleep because she was having terrifying nightmares. Ruth was reacting to the ordeal of the operation and trying to work through her experiences in her sleep. Possibly there were anaesthetic-induced dreams too. Medication and reassurances that she would be all right failed to ease Ruth's sleeping problems, so her mother and nursing staff worked together to solve the problem through play activities. She was encouraged to face the dream fears by imagining that there was another little girl coming into hospital. What could she do to help? She drew some pictures and made a small booklet to explain what would happen. She also played with special dolls, giving countless play injections, inserting and removing chest tubes and so on. Sometimes she played the doctor, sometimes the nurse, or even the patient. Within two days the nightmares disappeared.

After hospitalisation some children experience sleep disorders. It is not a subject that hospital staff tend to talk about, so parents are unprepared for the difficulties that arise. As part of the recuperation process listen to the child's dreams, let her talk out her fears or draw or play them. As Ruth's mother found, actively facing the fears dispels them, if it is done with love, sensitivity and patience.

Dream imagery in children with disabilities

Visual impairments

As a child Marjorie had a tendency towards nightmares and night terrors. Now a doctor, she understands why this was so: 'They may have arisen from my severe short-sightedness. As neither parent has this, they did not know that when I took my glasses off to go to bed, everything swelled and blurred and harmless objects could acquire a terrifying aspect.' These comments are worth bearing in mind if you have a short-sighted child.

Blind and disabled children dream about many of the same things that sighted children do. They dream of television characters and cartoons, of animals and family, of flying and wish-fulfilment delights, and they also have nightmares. They have dreams of illness as do their peers; however, their handicap has a definite influence on the nature of their dreams.

Children who lose their sight between the fifth and seventh years might still have visual images and REM periods during sleep, but if sight is lost before the fifth year there is no dream vision, as Joseph Jastrow noted as long ago as 1888. The congenitally blind cannot visualise. Usually they describe their dreams in tactile or auditory terms. My interviews with many young people at their school for visually impaired children confirmed this.

Shahzad (13) can see only in daylight. He told me:

> 'Last night I dreamt of a haunted house, saw vampires and ghosts. I panicked and fainted, then someone picked me up. I woke up and saw lots of vampires trying to turn me into a frog... I found magic books, I said *abracadabra* and *hocus pocus*, and changed the vampires. There were skeletons, I could hear their bones and chains rattling and the sound woke me up.'

Shahzad's basic self-confidence comes through in the dream, where in response to each threat he finds a means of escape. Shahzad tells his mother about his pleasant dreams. Usually she says 'very nice', but he protects her from other dreams because 'she doesn't like frightening things'. Another little girl at the school never talks to anyone about her dreams because 'they're special and they belong to me'. It is important to bear these comments in mind when talking to children about dreams, since they may have received all kinds of prescriptive messages that make it difficult to speak of their dream life. Respect for privacy is also very important, and no child should ever be pressured to reveal dreams they wish to keep secret.

Susan (8) has severe tunnel vision and can only see out of the corners of her eyes. She describes a disturbing dream:

> 'I dreamt about pulling my eye out. Mum put it in the bin and rubbish got on it. And then I went blind. She took it out and gave it to me, then I stuck it back in... Funny dream.'

Children do dream specifically of their visual handicap. Research reviewed by blind psychologist Donald Kirtley revealed that with adults, when blindness is the result of traumatic injury, there is much post-trauma dreaming as the dreamer comes to terms with what has happened. In some cases the action of the dreams proceeds up to the point just prior to the injury taking place, as if in her mind the dreamer stops the worst happening. Such dreams may continue for many years.

Javed (8) has heroic dreams of fighting for Robin and Batman against the Penguin, helping friends or foiling robbers. But he found one of his dreams particularly sad:

> 'Mum was going away because she didn't want to live at home any more. I followed them. Everyone (in the family) was going. Then they went to the motorway, then I got lost. They left me behind. There was no one to look after me.'

Javed is very dependent on those around him, particularly his family, and at times this arouses fears about what would happen if they should disappear. If dreams were 'on the agenda' and openly discussed, in the small tutorial groups at Javed's school for instance, there would be the opportunity to acknowledge and work through such widely shared fears.

Sounds are all important in the dreams of blind and partially sighted children. Jamie (3), an albino boy with severely restricted vision, generally likes dreaming and currently dreams of his dog fighting off a bad dragon. When I asked him how he knew his dog was there he told me he heard his loud growls. Similarly, Leon (9), blind from birth, relies on touch, smell, taste and movement to inform his dream world, and his dreams are vivid with sensation, texture and sound. His favourite dreams are full of gospel music, singing and clapping. Less warmly received is a dream of a witch who puts him on her back and flies on her broomstick. Sometimes the witch tries to eat him; he can feel and hear her.

Oscar (11) has cataracts, and was scared after *Jaws*. He said:

> 'I saw it in my head, the boat being smashed. I got killed. I get pictures in my head and eventually my brain doesn't want the picture so it eats it up. In my dreams my sight gets blurred and then I wake up.'

Other disabilities

REM sleep is specially important to infants, the neurologically impaired and those who have specific handicaps, such as autistic children. The brain continues to try to set down neural paths in dream sleep as a way of overcoming the handicap that inhibits effective learning. REM sleep may increase as part of the brain's attempt to cope with defects in the perceptual or motor systems.

As with visual impairment the range of dreams of deaf children depends on the extent of their disability. Daily events and personal relationships influence the dream content as with all children, but motor activity is of major importance. The critical period for auditory memory extends from the age of 3 to 7; deafness prior to age 3 usually results in muteness too, a factor that will be reflected in the child's dream life.

Helen Keller at 19 months contracted scarlet fever, which left her totally without sight, hearing, smell and speech. Aged 6 she began learning to communicate using the then popular finger alphabet. In 1904 she became the first deaf-blind person to receive a degree. In her book *The World I Live In* Helen Keller devoted two chapters to her dream life. She said she had sensations, aromas, tastes and ideas that she did not remember having experienced in waking reality. These may be remnants from infancy or intuitive knowledge. She found that her dreams were compensatory: in them she had greater physical freedom and more independence than in her waking life.

Whenever there has been 'normality' followed by sudden disability, physical or mental, dreams will attempt to come to terms with drastic changes imposed. Most research to date has been done with adults, but we have no reason to believe that the findings would not apply to children. For instance, Joseph Jastrow found that individuals who had undergone amputation of limbs in late childhood or as adults, continued to dream of themselves as physically whole for some time after the amputation. The 'phantom limb' remains in dreams.

As noted in Chapter 1, REM sleep is important for cognitive process. When a child has mental impairment or developmental delay there are difficulties with the mechanisms that enable learning to take place. According to Irwin Feinberg, in most instances REM sleep is severely curtailed when compared with non-handicapped children.

Ten-year-old George, who has Down's syndrome, was the only boy I came across who admitted to having wet dreams. These were about his girlfriend at school. Whether his candour was because he did not feel at all embarrassed about them I do not know. I do know that he found them enjoyable and much nicer than his frightening dreams about a snake! Perhaps the snakes were a more threatening aspect of his sexuality.

Psychological and emotional ill health

Of course, not all illness is physical. Some people suffering great emotional strain shared their dreams with me, and recurring themes were death and emotional pain. Harry now aged 14 told me how life was for him:

> 'When I was 13 I got put into care because my dad was on drugs and my mum was an alcoholic but then my mum got a job but I was in children's homes and with foster parents for a year. Last week I went back home and since I have been home I have been glue-sniffing and I have to talk to someone.'

On a good night he dreams that all will be well and he will be better soon. But more frequently his dreams are about being shot, his family being hurt and also being unable to move when he is being chased. Harry is stuck and feels powerless both in his dreams and with his family. His most frightening dream depicts with disturbing intensity a journey to the depths:

> 'I dreamt I was going down in the lift of the block of flats where I used to live. The lift would go down past the ground floor. Blood dripped out of the ventilator. The lift stopped and the door opened. Something was there but I couldn't see. I screamed but no sound came out.'

At the time of writing, Harry is back in the adolescent hospital unit, which will try to enable him to experience more positive ways of being in the world. This can be a monumental task when the emotional damage inflicted has been so destructive for such a long time; it is like learning to live all over again.

The British Psychological Society estimates that 10 per cent of children suffer mental illness serious enough to warrant treatment, as Michael Day in the *New Scientist* reported in 1997. Some children suffer distress in silence. Many of us will know children who seem to exist within a shroud of sorrow. Whether this is your own child or one you work with, it can feel particularly upsetting when you cannot ease the core of pain. We may never find out what it is that causes the unhappiness, yet we sense the desolation. What we do know is that there are significant numbers of young children who suffer from childhood depression.

Some children express distress through eating disorders as Janet Treasure (researcher and therapist at the Eating Disorders Unit, Bethlem and Maudsley Trust, London) describes in her book *Anorexia Nervosa: A Survival Guide for Families, Friends and Sufferers*. Children and young people suffering from anorexia nervosa sleep very little and lightly. This interferes with the pattern of dream (REM) sleep. However, when they start to eat more, they sleep more and more deeply and return once more to healing dream sleep.

If you are concerned about your child's mental health, listen to what he says about his dreams. If, allied to consistently distressing dreams, you see that your child is often tearful or sad, seems unable to make close relationships, has problems with eating and sleeping, and there have been major life stresses, such as moving house or illness, and you have a gut feeling that something is deeply amiss, then get help. Go to a sympathetic physician, find out if there are counselling services for young people in your area and get their support.

The REM state is influenced by personality disturbance, for instance in depression and psychosis. The eminent dream investigator Ernest Hartmann and his co-workers concluded, after considerable research in this area, that higher REM states happen in association with states of 'psychic pain', or at times of psychic imbalance when the dreamer attempts to change customary defence patterns. Thus quite often the person who requires more REM sleep is relatively anxious or depressed and there are changes in her life-style about which she worries. Nina (14), who lives in a professional middle-class family, is very happy most of the time. However, now and again she has mood swings, and the following nightmare came when she was quite depressed and sleeping for long periods:

> 'I dreamt that my mum and dad turned against me and wouldn't let me into the house. All my friends had turned against me. I was all alone. I started crying and then I killed myself.'

American sleep researcher Ernest Rossi argues that this need for increased REM sleep is because of chemico-biological changes which are occurring in the brain as proteins are synthesised.

Leonard Handler, an American therapist, described the way he worked with an 11-year-old boy diagnosed as emotionally disturbed and minimally brain-damaged. For about a year and a half John had been having terrifying nightmares: he would wake up in a panic and rush to his parents' room. The monster in his dreams chased him and sometimes caught and hurt him. In order to ease the situation Handler, who had developed a good rapport with the boy, used confrontation therapy. Using this method the child was asked to sit on the therapist's knee, thus providing physical proximity and security. Then, having been reassured that they would fight the monster together, the boy was asked to close his eyes and visualise it. When he said he could see it, the therapist held him more closely while pounding on the desk and shouting something to the effect: 'Get away from my friend you lousy monster! If you come back I'll be with John and we'll fight you.' This was repeated a number of times, with John eventually feeling empowered to join in the 'seeing-off' of the monster. When asked in the next session whether he had seen the monster, John replied that he had but had yelled at it and it had disappeared. Six months later the nightmares had still not returned. This fantasy technique can be used by adults who have a strong trusting relationship with a child.

Abuse

Children who are abused often deal with the abuse in their dreams. Incest victims suffer nightmares or other sleep disorders, as psychologist Alice Miller describes in *Breaking Down the Wall of Silence*. Many abused children feel utterly distraught and confused. The confusion arises in part because they see an adult as an authority figure and yet they have been forced to do something wrong by that authority. So somehow the action must be all right. At a gut level, victims feel it is wrong, but they cannot argue against the emotional and physical pressure put on them by the abuser. Many nightmares will reflect severe anxiety about being chased, perhaps by big, heavy creatures such as elephants, and being powerless and unable to escape. The element of force is predominant. While many children have anxiety dreams about being pursued by an anonymous stranger, abused children are much more likely to dream of the actual molester. The chief emotion in the dreams is helplessness.

Patricia Garfield, in her study of the dreams of sexually abused girls, found that their dream life differs in many ways from those of non-abused children. Being chased figured in over 50 per cent of their dreams, but, most significantly, the chase ended in an attack on the dreamer. Not only was there attack but it usually resulted in the death of the dreamer, the mother or a younger sibling. This is not surprising, since the dreamer had been subject to actual attacks when awake. Dream death, then, is a common outcome.

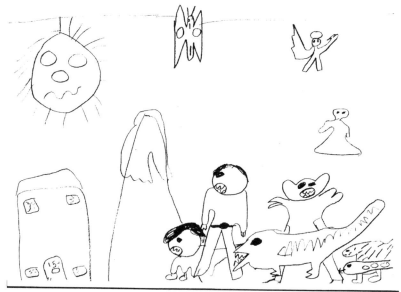

Danger All Around

Children who are sexually abused are frequently told by the abuser that they will be killed if they tell anyone of their abuse. Sometimes they are told that by complying they are 'saving' a younger sibling from a similar attack. All too often, abused children feel as if part of themselves has been murdered; their right to make choices about their own body has been taken away and their trust has been killed. Dreams tell us of these feelings.

When Bernadette was 10 she used to dream of being attacked by a bull. Though her sister was there, she did nothing to save Bernadette. She also dreamt of being held prisoner in an underground cell. She described her childhood: 'My home was broken. My sisters and I were battered, there were constant rows, very little money. We had to stay upstairs out of the way. At the time I did not think I was unhappy.' Now she realises just how damaging her experiences were. Her early abusive experiences scarred her emotionally. Intimate, trusting relationships, now she is an adult, are immensely difficult. For children who receive supportive therapy this need not be the outcome.

Child-abuse statistics make grim reading. Research by Ellen Bass and Louise Thornton, American authors and writing workshop leaders, indicates that one in four girls and one in seven boys will be sexually abused by the age of 12. This means that most of us will come in contact with someone – family, friend, neighbour, colleague – who has suffered abuse. If you are concerned with the welfare of children, listen to their dreams when they share them and be alert to signals they send. As Lord Justice Butler-Sloss said in her report on the Cleveland Inquiry, there are not enough people listening to what children say.

Jean Goodwin of the University of New Mexico Department of Psychiatry described how drawings of dreams are used both to ascertain the nature of the abuse and to enable the child to work through the damaging experiences she has been subject to. One 9-year-old girl drew a dream picture of herself in a wedding dress standing in front of a house in a field full of flowers. She talked to the therapist about her dream, and spoke of her longing for a new father and a new marriage for her mother, and of her fear that her mother would not be able to divorce the father who had committed incest. Goodwin commented on the fact that flowers may be used symbolically by girls who feel 'de-flowered', as in this dream. She had worked with one very depressed and abused 7-year-old, who drew page after page of drooping flowers that had been stripped of their petals.

Jan, now in her forties, told me of a recurring dream she had from the age of 9 to 12:

> 'I was in a vast dark hall. The floor was white and black squares like a chessboard and there were four staircases, one in each corner, going nowhere. Light came from above like a dull spotlight. At the top of each stairway stood a man in robes – no faces visible. I was thrown from one figure to the other, not necessarily aggressively but each time I was not confident I would be caught. Each figure held me briefly and passed me on. No sound.'

The dream began after she was first subjected to sadistic sexual abuse, which was repeated over a period of time. You can see how the imagery of the dream symbolically discloses her feelings of being a 'pawn' in a game in which she has no say, nor any power. She withdraws into soundless isolation, no one is there to take her part. As is often the case, it is too dangerous to acknowledge the faces of these figures who can toss her about so casually. She is completely at their mercy and at any moment may be indifferently 'dropped' to her destruction.

Children who have explicit dreams involving a repetition of the sexual activity that constitutes the abuse, will very rarely describe such dreams unless they have found a safe, non-judgemental environment in which to do so. Threats from the abuser should the 'secret' be revealed cause such dreams to be feared and censored to the outside world. And children for years have been disbelieved when they spoke of abuse. Since Freud's rejection of his first findings on the high incidence of sexual abuse, when he chose to view the experiences revealed to him as fantasy rather than fact, a legacy of disbelief has been the lot of too many children. It is vital now that we do not betray children again by denying the terrible problems of their abuse.

Terminal illness

Dr Elisabeth Kübler-Ross, famous for her work with those who are terminally ill, found that most children know what is happening to them and go through the same common grieving patterns as adults. They too experience denial, anger, bargaining, depression and acceptance. Acceptance involves an awareness of the situation and a determination to live life to its fullest in their remaining days. Fear will also be very much at the forefront of a child's experience of facing death, and dreams often reflect their deepest anxieties. Kübler-Ross found that children symbolically express their knowledge of death to those who will hear them. So it is vitally important for us to listen to the dreams that they try to tell us. They are an important part of the process of 'letting go'.

In terminal illness, patients often dream of death when others may be trying to keep the truth about their condition from them. However, it is important to recognise that dreams of death in the healthy or slightly ill person are much more to do with the expression of fears about dying or about the 'death' of one aspect of life and the 'birth' of another. For instance, many adults dream of the death of a partner around the time of divorce. Such dreams reflect emotional changes rather than physical death.

Where children have a life-threatening illness, nightmares and night terrors may develop. A 3-year-old girl who was diagnosed with acute leukaemia began to have both and was so distressed that she needed further paediatric care. The nightmares began when she was separated from her mother on her admission for treatment and when the invasive treatment was administered. These nightmares alerted her family and physicians to the severe anxiety she was unable to express when she was awake. American pediatrician Jonathan Kellerman describes how reassurance and anxiety reduction were central to her health care.

Dreams prior to illness, during illness and following illness can help us to understand how our minds and bodies are working. They may reveal the way in which some of us have an underlying need for symptoms, a covert need to be ill in order to avoid stressful situations or to give ourselves a break from stressful lives. In neurotic and psychosomatic illnesses, which are as debilitating and painful as organic illnesses, self-enlightenment aids healing. Learning about dreams can help both children and adults develop insightful, health-promoting self-awareness.

Dreams at this time often act as a connection to a further dimension, a spiritual world where other laws seem to operate.

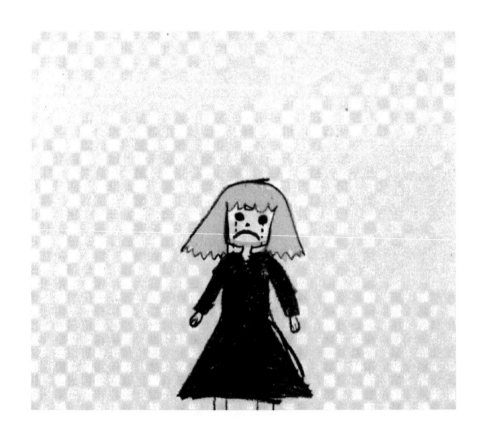

Sad Child

Chapter Nine

Worlds Torn Apart
Loss and Conflict

The matrix which makes dreams in us has been called an inner spiritual guide, an inner centre of the psyche. Most primitive people just called it God, or a god. The highest god of the Aztecs, for instance, was the maker of dreams and guided people through their dreams.

Marie-Louise von Franz in Fraser Boa's *The Way of the Dream*

Separation from loved ones, divorce, loss and death are part of a child's experience of life and they affect their dreams. In this chapter we focus on how we can use dreams to help the child deal with their loss and discover how dreams can re-connect us to people who have died.

Separation and divorce

Divorce is one of the most serious crises in Western contemporary life. Though most members of a divorced family ultimately cope with and come to terms with this critical life event, psychologist Judith Wallerstein and her colleagues Sandra Blakeslee and Julia Levis in their book *The Unexpected Legacy of Divorce: A 25 Year Landmark Study* show us that there is no such thing as a victimless divorce.

'When I went to the fair and my mum and dad had an argument
and my mum walked away and they had a divorce.'

Kerry (9)

Kerry said this was her most frightening dream. At the back of her mind
was the niggling worry that her mother and father were about to split up.
No one had spoken of it, yet she could not bring herself to ask any direct
questions in case she caused trouble and got blamed.

In the midst of parental conflict, children worry about the break-up of
their home, having to choose who to live with, what will happen to the
parent who moves out and what will happen about school. Often they
think that somehow it is their fault that the relationship between their
parents went wrong. They blame themselves and develop guilt feelings,
which can lead to disturbed and self-destructive behaviour.

Aaron (12) told me that he has 'great parents', whom he loves very
much, yet he dreams of:

'...my parents splitting up and it is me who takes all the pain of
who I want to go with and what would happen.'

He can talk to his parents about most of his frightening dreams, and they
are usually able to calm his nerves. But somehow this one, which expresses
one of his worst fears, he cannot share with them. Other children's dreams
act as preparation for events to come. This is similar to the 'rehearsal'
dreams we saw in Chapter 7.

It is clear from these dreams that children do worry about parents' separating. Now, in response to such stress, there is more research going into
conciliation and mediation processes. With the help of a neutral, trained
mediator, issues of custody, access and ongoing support for the children, as
well as the financial arrangements are dealt with. Apart from the saving in
legal fees, families are helped to communicate with each other at a time
when anger and resentment may make it otherwise impossible.

'I dream that my dad pushed me and my sister and my mum over
the edge of a cliff and we're all falling.'

Jennifer (9)

Falling is the main theme of her dream, which Jennifer recognised was
provoked by her parents' struggle during their violent pre-separation

period. In waking life she feels she is going 'over the edge' because she cannot control what is going on in her life. It reflects her belief that she has no secure ground left in her family life. When I asked her how she was feeling, she replied: 'It's hard with my family falling apart. Now my dad has gone and one of the best parts of my family, my nan, has died.' Her one solid landmark in the shifting ground was her constant, loving grandmother and her death was an additional loss Jennifer had to face.

If you are involved in separating from or divorcing a partner you will find that talking to your children and answering their questions is ultimately the most constructive approach you can take. Even if you do not know what the outcome will be, you can prevent the build-up of fearful fantasies that the children resort to in order to fill gaps in their knowledge. If a child has facts from you, and your ideas about what may happen in the future, he is less likely to assume it will be a nightmare.

Moving out

Many children express distress in their dreams that they keep hidden during waking life. Karoline Proksch and Michael Schredl, who looked at the dreams of children whose parents had divorced, found that their dreams contained more unsuccessful roles. Emma's (8) father recently left home and it affected her dreams:

> 'I dream about bad people coming to take me away. But my sister, Kelly, she dreams a lot of nightmares that get her sleepwalking. She sleepwalks outside. We both dream about men coming to take us away. We had the same dream on the same night.'

She feels that at any moment she may be 'removed' from home and there is no one to protect her or her sister.

Sally's parents split up recently, and now she has recurring dreams about her 'dad being in the house on his own'. Her other distressing dreams reflect further anxiety about the separation; in the worst one she dreams her parents are dying. She is so disturbed that she cannot go back to sleep afterwards.

For some children separation and divorce can be a welcome relief from a warring partnership. For Paula (12) there are no romantic images of the Father Christmas-like absent father who turns up once a week bearing gifts; she is happier living in a loving, stable, single-parent household. In her most frightening dream, she says, 'My real dad came back and was going to take me away.' She is afraid of being used as a pawn in a game that her father might play with her mother. Children are often used a pawns in matrimonial conflict, and confusion may arise in the child who feels forced to reject, or protect, one parent in favour of another. We see the ensuing anxiety in disturbing dreams, problem behaviour and poor schoolwork.

Torn loyalties

Many children have dreams that feature the new partner of their parent. In some cases the child feels torn between liking the new partner and not wanting to feel that he is letting his 'missing' parent down. Separation has been repeated many times in Leigh's short life. Now 12 years old, she continues to have a disturbing cluster of dreams:

> 'I dream of people murdering me or my family. When I'm ill I dream that the doctors give me the wrong medicine and I die. In another one I was in a big factory and it was very scary. I was even crying in my sleep and I can feel this man stabbing me when I am sleeping. And I wake up crying. I go into the bathroom and wash my face and I think the dream will go away but it doesn't.'

Her nights are filled with hideous dreams. When I spoke to her she confided that two of her baby brothers had died and her mother and father split up. She said: 'I don't see that that [the deaths] has anything to do with the dreams. It's just my mum, she's forbidden me to talk about it at home or anywhere. Sometimes I feel I'll burst. I just don't know what to do.'

Children who are part of a divorcing family feel a deep sense of loss. They often feel a profound sense of emptiness, grief, an inability to concentrate and fatigue, and have troublesome dreams; all are symptoms of mourning. As J. William Worden, former professor of psychology at Harvard Medical School, points out, although no one has died, they mourn the death of the family of their childhood. Small children in particular need someone reliable to whom they can turn when distressed or threatened. If this security base disappears, as in separation, then the child becomes more vulnerable and needs support in order to build up his own inner security.

Bereavement

When a parent dies

Bruce (8) dreams of his father who died 'a long time ago'; but the dreams don't comfort him, they make him sad. He talks to his brother about his dreams, but his mother won't listen to them because she does not like it when he mentions his father. Where this happens, children like Bruce cannot grieve, they cannot go through the process of mourning and letting go.

Sometimes in Bruce's dreams, aliens from space come down and eat him up. I told Bruce that I would find that a frightening dream; I empathised with his discomfort and he revealed that he was being bullied at school. The devouring aliens symbolise the boys who bully him, they are 'alien' to him. Their boisterous extroversion is the antithesis of his bowed reticence. There is no one, at school or at home, to whom Bruce can talk because he believes no one wants to listen. If you want to help a child like Bruce, listen; it is one of the most valuable helping skills there is.

A child whose relationship with a caring parent has been wounded, through whatever cause, may become preoccupied with self, become someone who shows off or who always has to win at everything. This may be a form of compensation that could appear in dreams.

Bringing them back in dreams

Children come to terms with death in all sorts of ways. Some believe that after death the dead person will come alive again. Partly this is to do with watching television programmes where the almost-dead rise in time for the next episode, and partly to do with beliefs about life after death. Eight-year-old Mel's recurring dream shows how she reacted to the death of her cousin and how long the grieving process can take:

> 'I used to dream of my cousin who was four years old when she died and very close to me. After her death I dreamt that she woke me up and we used to play with her dolls. I was always depressed

after that dream. I always wanted to die, wishing I could die so I could live with her and play with her. I always played with her in my dreams, for a year after she died and occasionally now in my dreams I have visions of walking up steps and meeting her and we would go and see Santa Claus. Sometimes I still wish I could live with her.'

Jungian psychoanalyst Marie-Louise von Franz found in her extensive work on dreams of death that dreaming of the deceased facilitates the grieving process; the deceased returns to life allowing the past and present to be integrated, and this enables the dreamer to complete the process so she can attain closure.

Death of a significant person in life is a devastating experience for children. One of the ways we make up for the physical loss may be by imagining the person who has died and, as an extension of this, dreaming that the loved one is with us once more. Stuart (12) does this:

'I dream that my grandad, who's dead, sits at the end of my bed and sings to me.'

Deborah, though very upset when her grandfather died, found solace in a dream where he told her that he was happy and well and that Deborah and the rest of the family need not be upset. The dream released her, it gave her permission to finish grieving and move forward in her life.

During their development children naturally experience a stage where they have fears, often at bedtime, that their parents will die. Such fears and dreams can be terrifying. It is very distressing for adults too. To sit and comfort a child who says 'Mummy, you're not going to die are you? You won't die will you?' is painful because it forces you to face the fact that you might die before your child grows up. There are no guarantees for any of us. We have to find ways of reassuring our children and empowering them emotionally so that they can cope with loss.

Maxwell (9) told me about his dream:

'In my dream all the family was at the crematorium. My grandad had died. The coffin was just about to disappear behind the curtains. The vicar was just saying, "Now Sidney G— is to be cremated." Just then there came a croaking noise from the coffin.

It started to open and Grandad got out of it. And after that every-thing was all right.'

Maxwell's mother added: 'On the third night after grandad died, my husband too had a similar dream to Maxwell's. He dreamt there was a knock on the door and the doctor appeared with my husband's dad. He said they'd taken Grandad to hospital and that they'd removed something from his throat and that he was perfectly all right. Both my husband and Maxwell rarely remember their dreams, but this dream woke them and they were able to recall it. The next day we talked about the dreams and Grandad's death at length. Maxwell said that he knew Grandad was now happy in heaven with Granny, he just wished he was still with us.'

Maxwell is fortunate to have a mother who is willing to talk about death. Charles Darwin, great scientific explorer and pioneer of his genera-tion, suffered throughout his life from chronic ill health. From the evidence available it is clear that his poor health was psychiatric and psy-chosomatic in origin. His mother died when he was only 9 years old, and two of his three sisters would not allow his mother's name ever to be men-tioned. Darwin himself in later years said he could remember nothing about her at all. The overwhelming taboo drove his pain into the darkness of the unconscious; its only expression was through continued illness. In dreams, death very often symbolises the ending of one phase of life and the beginning of another.

Anticipation of loss

Children think and dream about death quite frequently. Often they are prompted by waking events such as the death of a pet, a television programme or a book. Helen (10) had been reading *Tom's Midnight Garden* at school, which is one trigger for the dream, but in addition, she told me:

'I was sleeping at my Gran's house, which is filled with war relics – medals, letters and photographs. I dreamt I was a soldier in the Second World War. Me and lots of other soldiers are in a wintry forest. All the trees are bare and there is snow on the ground. It's cold and I'm wearing a large trenchcoat. We are all running away from German soldiers who are firing guns at us. I get shot and fall down. The last thing I say is "Please God, don't let me die".'

Gretta (10) found a ladybird. Wanting to keep it as a pet, she put it in a matchbox, as many children do, but it died. When her sister then died suddenly, disturbing dreams troubled Gretta. She dreamt that huge, slug-like creatures were climbing up the outside wall of her house and into her bedroom. She had recurring dreams of rows upon rows of grey crosses in an endless cemetery. Nothing happened other than the defeating repetition of gravestones continuing into infinity.

These dreams include a number of common features found in dreams connected with death. At a simple level there is Gretta's guilt at killing the harmless ladybird that she wanted to keep. Her dream invaders are creepy-crawlies too and are out to wreak revenge, as it appears to a sensitive 10-year-old. Then there is the enormity of her sister's death; Gretta suddenly learns that death goes on and on, thousands upon thousands of dream headstones reiterate the truth she has had to face. Her dreams are part of the processing of her trauma. The dream enables her to contemplate a powerful truth. It is a way for her psyche to give her space to consider and reflect. In the fast pace of many children's lives there is little time to sit and think.

Gretta's slug dream also mirrors her waking thoughts about being eaten by worms and fearful fantasies she had had about her sister's burial and its consequences. Her dreams allowed expression of thoughts. If a child asks 'Will worms eat her?', she is usually shushed and told not talk like that. The thoughts do not go away but have to be dealt with in some way; the dreaming process allows this to take place.

Sudden death

Grieving is a necessary part of responding to death in a healthy way. It is normal to have a wide range of responses to death: to feel sorrow; to feel anger, perhaps at being left behind to cope with ongoing problems; to feel guilt, perhaps because we feel we should have done more. These reactions are to be expected. Where death has been unexpected or in unusual circumstances, however, grieving can be a much more problematic experience. American art therapist Felice Cohen (1978) records her work with a little boy, Mark, whose brother had died in a fire inadvertently started by both boys. Mark was referred to her for therapy two years after the fire. At that time he had a range of problematic symptoms: he ate compulsively, hit and bit himself and provoked fights with family and friends. He seemed constantly to seek out punishment. The situation was becoming intolerable.

Mark's parents did not openly grieve, and their son was ignored and left unconsoled; understandably they found their own ambivalent feelings towards their remaining son extremely difficult. Felice says that after four months of painting pictures he began to accompany his drawings with descriptions of his tormented dreams in which red-hot fires consumed him. He asked why he had not been allowed to go to the funeral, why his parents would not talk to him about Scotty, and asked why he too could not have died. That was the turning point in his therapy. No one had ever explained what had happened, no one had ever used the word 'accident' in reference to the tragedy. Stuck in his mind was the image that Scotty was taken away and no one ever mentioned him again. After a further three months in art therapy, working through his grief and realising that he had not murdered his brother, Mark's original problems were resolved. He and his parents were able to be more open emotionally and were able to share as a family once more.

What can we tell the children?

Very young children taste grief. Psychiatrist John Bowlby (1985) concluded, in his work on attachment and loss in children's lives, that children as young as 15 months experienced loss in the same way as adults. They go through the four common stages of mourning; an initial numbness with occasional bouts of intense anger or distress, then searching and yearning for the lost person, disorganisation and despair, and finally, if all goes well, there is a reconciliation and acceptance of the loss. This grieving process of denial, anger, guilt and acceptance may last for many months; commonly two years is needed. It is wrong to believe that children rapidly forget about death, they do not. So allow time and be patient.

As we have seen, children dream about death and they think about it. Telling them not to worry about it does not help. From an early age children need honesty and simple, straightforward explanations. If the death has been of a parent, there is the added burden that the remaining parent may be so upset herself that she cannot cope with the child's grief as well. Just when the child needs most stability and parental love, he may be sent away to relatives and have additional separation to deal with, without the security of his usual environment. Children need to work through their own pain and loss without being made to feel guilty about it. To grieve as a family is a powerfully healing experience.

Variations on a theme

There are all sorts of loss that children experience. Moving house or country brings huge changes in a child's life and by working with dreams you can help the child to express their feelings. Before Helen (11) moved house she had several dreams about what it would be like.

> 'In my dreams I invented people, but all my old friends were there as well.'

She said she still dreams about her old and new friends mixed together, even though it is seven months since she relocated. Adjusting to a new place takes time, and a different accent may make it even harder for some children to be accepted in the new school community.

> 'Sometimes, I dream I am going back to Iraq on an aeroplane and some men take the plane and kill me.'
>
> Bashar (11)

Loss may be of a country as well as of a person. Bashar, an Iraqi boy who lived in England temporarily, said, 'I dream I go back to my country and me and my friends, we do a party.' This dream combined fear with wish-fulfilling elements of going home; tied in with his loss of roots was his fear of what might happen if he were to return to the war zone.

Dreams are likely to become more disturbing at times when a child leaves one school to move on to the next stage in his education. All change is stressful and children develop fears and have anxious thoughts about the new situation that awaits them. Listening to worries, providing information, and familiarisation with the new school all help alleviate their fears. Pay attention to dream narratives, for they will tell you a lot about how your child is settling down. If he is not adjusting successfully, then disturbing dreams and sleep problems may become exacerbated.

The impact of war

Children dream of war

A weapon is an enemy even to its owner.

Turkish proverb

Since 1945 there has not been a single day on which the world has been at peace. Armed conflicts have raged somewhere on earth: Vietnam, Mozambique, South Africa, Lebanon, Ireland, the Falklands, Bosnia. On September 11 2001, the World Trade Centre attack left America and the world reeling. Both children and adults, traumatised by what they had experienced directly or watched on television, reported an increase in disturbing dreams and nightmares. In direct response to this the Association for the Study of Dreams set up a 24 hour helpline to offer support. When the world seems turned upside down children's dreams reflect their terror. What effect does this have on children now?

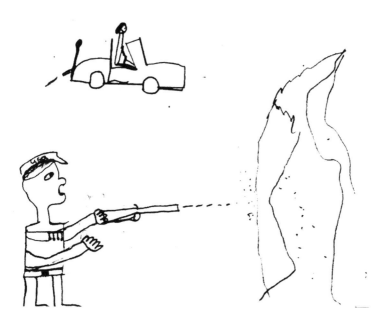

Boy with USA cap and gun

Play is vitally important to a child's development; indeed, as Dr Donald Winnicott, perhaps the greatest English psychoanalyst, famed for his work with children said, 'play is the work of childhood'. Through play, children express their knowledge of the world and attempt to master it. Through play, they practise skills. However, what we see in places of armed conflict such as Albania, Palestine and Israel is that children play at war, at being terrorists and gunmen, they play at being strong and in control, they play at having power when they are powerless. In their play with their toys children are assertive rather than passive, which is a healthy progression. In working with children's war dreams we can use them as a basis of play and conflict resolution. Be directed by the child rather than telling her what to do. That way you will discover much more about how she sees the world.

Many children who lived through the worst of the conflict in Northern Ireland found that their dreams mirrored this. Their dreams were of terrorists, gunmen, funerals and war. Nichola (12), whose uncle was killed in the horrific Milltown Cemetery attack in Belfast, dreamt:

> 'When we had only just moved into our house and we were unpacking, I was upstairs putting my toys away when I heard a gun shot and saw a man with a gun in our backyard, so I ran downstairs and told my mammy and daddy. They went out the back and saw nothing but later that night when my mammy was putting up curtains she saw a man with blood all over his face at the window. He shouted "Nichola, Nichola!", but it was my mammy waking me up for school.'

The blood-streaked dream man is seeking Nichola and she is afraid. At first her parents cannot see this intruder as perhaps they cannot see just how terrified she sometimes feels in waking life. She recognised that one of the reasons we dream is to relieve anxiety. She commented: 'We need to dream to sort out a problem or because we have something on our minds which causes us to have stress and we have to think it over.'

10-year-old Emma's father was shot one night as he was walking home in the Ardoyne district of Belfast. She dreamt:

> 'Once I dreamt about a man who was a member of the army, who got blew up right in front of my eyes. Then I got shot three times

in the eyes so I couldn't identify the person who blew the soldier up.'

A terrifying picture of a child innocently witnessing a horrific act, yet in her dream she also becomes a victim. Many children's dreams expressed fear of paramilitary groups, from either side of the sectarian divide. Like many children living in conditions of war, they know that very little special consideration will be given because they are children.

Children need time to describe their nightmares and to be reassured that they are not alone, bad or mad because they have disturbing dreams. Children need help in understanding that nightmares are symptomatic of the stress under which they live. Mastering their experiences through dream-work is another useful tool in the emotional-repair work kit. In Haifa, psychologist Ofra Ayalon works with Israeli children in classrooms, helping them to cope with their anxieties. By understanding the original traumatic events or those which may arise, such as air raids and bombings, children may no longer be overwhelmed. Although they still feel sad, they share fears and are not trapped in isolating fear. They can more easily cope with living.

Dreams about war come from many sources: from stories children hear from grandparents, from films, from history lessons at school, from the news they watch on television. They learn of war and experience fear. Those who live in war zones actually live the terror their dreams portray.

Ruth (10) dreamt that Russia and America had a fight and they blew up the whole world. She drew a child calling 'Help' and a sad-faced woman shouting 'Where are my children?' Another figure with tears flowing to the floor says 'We are all going to die'. Ruth said everyone would be killed and no one would be alive after this war. Ruth has no direct, personal experience of war, though she is affected by it.

Personal experience of war makes a profound impact. In a study, commissioned by Prince Talal bin Abdul-Aziz, it was found that more than 58 per cent of Lebanese children are suffering from stress-related illnesses because of the civil war there. Children nearer home suffer similar stress and this is reflected in the dreams of children in conflict-scarred Northern Ireland.

> 'My most frightening dreams are about bombs. I have never had a happy dream.'

James (7)

Orla from Belfast was 11 when she had this dream which was influenced by the sectarian conflict in which she lived:

> 'I dreamt that I woke up to go to the toilet and I heard a ticking noise downstairs. I went down and realised it was a bomb. I started screaming and woke everybody up. They all came downstairs and got out of the house before it blew up.'

The Northern Irish children I interviewed for my research and those I filmed for the BBC documentary 'Children Dreaming', no matter which 'side' they belonged to, had worrying dreams about being hurt. Shauna (9)'s comment is typical:

> 'I normally dream about the IRA breaking into our house and I hide behind the cupboard so that if they killed everyone else they wouldn't get me.'

The threat of nuclear war

Dr Eric Chivian, staff psychiatrist at the Massachusetts Institute of Technology, writing in *The Human Cost of Nuclear War*, found in his study of American children's knowledge of and response to nuclear issues that children absorbed messages of anxiety and despair from their culture. One 7-year-old girl said that she wished she could go to heaven and not have to worry about 'all this stuff about nuclear war'.

Margaret (11), who attends a primary school in England, had this dream:

> 'Once I dreamt that nuclear war broke out and Ireland was blown up and my family and I were all on different parts of the world and I was just floating on a very, very small plot of land. The rest of the world had sunk under the sea.'

She was able to wake to her mother's reassuring voice, but how easy is it to be comforting, especially if you live in the shadow of a nuclear power station and your child attends a school in which a store of anti-radiation pills are kept 'just in case' there is an accident?

Racism

In her diary Anne Frank wrote of her nocturnal dreams and her intense desire for peace. She was eventually put to death in Belsen concentration camp. In Terezin concentration camp near Prague, where fifteen thousand children were deported, we see the harrowing outcome of extreme racism. Like Anne Frank, the children of Terezin wrote about their dreams and drew pictures of them because dreams gave them an escape from their waking misery. (Green 1978)

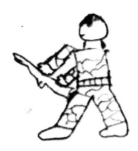

A number of children recalled dreams of the Holocaust, Jews and non-Jews alike. Paul (11) explained:

> 'The most frightening dream I had was fighting a war with Germany and I was put in a chamber of gas.'

Hannah (12), a member of a flourishing Jewish youth group, said that her most frightening dream was when she was caught up in the Holocaust and was in a concentration camp. After studying *The Diary of Anne Frank* in literature classes other children found their dreams peopled with her characters.

Many children suffer racial abuse. For example, Najwa (10), born in England of Pakistani parents, has suffered many verbal assaults and numerous threatened physical attacks:

'My most frightening dream was, I was riding my bike and my daddy was sweeping the garden and this man was being nasty to this boy so my daddy started to tell him off, but he just kicked him and then he came and took me away.'

Shaista's nightmare, told to me after a number of fire attacks on the homes of Asians had been reported in the press, reveals her fears that she does not speak about:

'I had to light a fire to my house when everybody was asleep because two people came in and thought my dad was a bank manager and they wanted to rob the bank without my dad finding out, so they told me to light fire to my house, but I didn't and they lit fire for me.'

Shaista (11)

The import of these dreams is clear. Children are deeply affected by the wars they are forced to live with. And while external conflict rages, we need to bear in mind that these children have the same internal wars raging as children everywhere. From infancy to adolescence they struggle to learn, to become independent and to become self-directed individuals. But, whatever happens, dreams will encompass and reveal the process and progress of our children's lives.

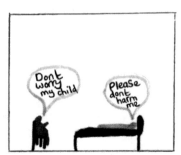 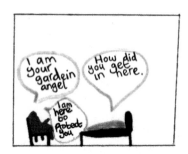

This Story is about a dream
I had about my gaurdein angel was
coming to my bed in the night
to protect me through the
night.

Guardian Angel

Chapter Ten

Guiding Lights
The Spiritual Dimension of Dreams

For the Tikopians [a people from Polynesia] the dream is an adventure of the spirit. Dream experience, in fact, is taken as evidence of the spirit world to which everyone has access. The dream is a creation of the spirit world, being the outcome of what is enacted there.

Carl W. O'Neill, *Dreams, Culture, and the Individual*

Dreams have played a part in all major religious traditions. They have been, and still are, used as a means of exploring unseen realms usually inaccessible in waking life.

Divine origins

Buddhists believe, as do adherents to so many other religious traditions, that certain dreams have divine origins. Robert van der Castle, the former director of the Sleep and Dream Laboratory at the University of Virginia Medical School, in *Our Dreaming Mind* tells how the mother of the Buddha dreamt that four kings carried her bed to the top of a mountain where four queens greeted her with jewels and took her to a golden palace. Then an elephant with six ivory tusks appeared and painlessly pierced her side. When she woke she realised she had conceived and that her child would be a world leader or a world teacher.

Hear now my words: If there be a prophet among you, I the Lord
will make myself known to him in a vision, and will speak to him
in a dream.

Num. 12:6

Christianity also places a high significance on dream revelations. The Bible
has more than twenty references to divine guidance, some of which
changed the course of history. In working with children's dreams it is
helpful to demonstrate just how important dreams have been throughout
history.

The flight into Egypt is linked to three dreams: the first is the dream of
the wise men who are warned not to return to Herod, the second is the one
in which an angel warns the Holy Family to go to Egypt to escape from
Herod, and the third which tells Joseph he can return to Israel because
Herod is dead. The dream of Pontius Pilate's wife however, was not
heeded. On the day of the crucifixion she begged her husband to free Jesus
rather than Barabbas because of a dream she had about him.

St John Crysostom (CE 347–407) preached about the importance of
dreams and said they were a link to the divine. He also said that we are not
responsible for our dreams so we should not be ashamed of the images and
actions that take place in dreams. His mother who dreamt of his conversion
to Christianity nine years before it took place may have sparked off St
Augustine's interest in dreams.

In many cultures no division was made between visions and divine
messages that came in dreams. Mohammed received spiritual instructions
in both states. The Prophet had his first revelation in a dream and knew he
had to found the new religion of Islam. His most important dream, known
as the Night Journey, initiated him into the mysteries of the cosmos.

Religious influences

Dreams generally reflect the religious upbringing the child has experienced. As you might expect they can be comforting or disturbing as these
two dreams show:

'I flew away to a desert island with my two sisters and the king of
the sea came and lifted the island and brought us to heaven. There

were angels flying and at the gate of heaven I saw angels welcoming me in.'

Sean (11)

'My mummy told me not to go near this house but I didn't do as I was told. When I went in the door jammed. A big demon appeared – he wanted my soul. Then I woke up shouting 'You're not getting it!'

Eamon (11)

Some people say 'The bogey man will get you', but Eamon has learnt that the devil will get him if he does not do as he is told. Parents sometimes use threats to make children conform; but beware, such fears can get out of control and severely disturb developing minds, for children may take you literally and believe that devils stalk them. That applies to Violet (11), a Catholic girl from Belfast, who dreamt that the devil appeared at the end of her bed and told her he would not go back to hell without her.

'My worst nightmare was when my friend Carole knocked at my door and I answered and she turned into a demon. My daddy came down and got the sledgehammer and knocked her over the head with it. Then she turned into a dog and I kept her.'

Cara (13)

In this dream Cara's father can control the evil that is present. He protects her and so she can keep this friend/animal that she had doubts about. Whether it is her friend she has misgivings about or a projection of her own 'demonic' qualities on to the friend, she will be all right finally because her father is in control: she can rely on him.

Coming to terms with heaven and earth can be a painful process as 13-year-old Daniel related: 'My most frightening dream was that I died and I found there was no heaven.'

Peak or transcendental experiences

'Talking to God is like being on the telephone, you can't see him but you know he's listening.'

Mina (7)

According to Edward Robinson in *The Original Vision*, most, if not all, people are capable of having 'peak experiences' as the American psychologist Abraham Maslow terms them. This means that children too have experiences which go beyond their everyday world and connect them to something outside the ordinary and rational. For some children this can be quite disturbing, especially if adults tell them the experience or the dream is nonsense.

In 'peak experiences' time and space are suspended. The person experiences a oneness with the universe, a heightened sense of intrinsic values such as truth, beauty and joy. The importance of the physical world diminishes and self is transcended: we 'know' we are more than the physical body we inhabit. Such transcendent, peak experiences are often linked to religious experience, though not exclusively. Many adults can remember these feelings from age four or five, so they are not only the province of the grown-up world. Children you come in contact with may well have transcendent experiences but have not had the opportunity to share them. Working with dreams can be a powerful way to introduce this spiritual dimension. As such, it helps the child be open to the possibility of experiencing the divine in mysterious ways.

> 'My happiest dream was when I was in a garden. It was sunny. I was at a gate and went through it and there was a man, very old, saying "Go back, you've a lifetime before you come through here".'
>
> Vicky (10)

When Vicky had this dream she felt she'd been to heaven, or on the verge of it, and was filled with joy tinged with sadness. She had wanted to stay in the sublime space with this wise old man, yet knew that it would always be there for her and that sometime in the future she would return to it.

> 'My best dream was about me and God.'
>
> Anthony (10)

Life after death

> 'When my grandfather died I dreamed he came to say "Goodnight" and "Goodbye".'
>
> William (8)

Dreams of people who are dying often involve reference to life after death. Marie-Louise von Franz, a Jungian analyst who has completed extensive research with people approaching death, says that their dreams can be interpreted as preparation for the deep transformation that it brings and for the continuation of life after death. I explore this in depth in my book *Dreams, Counselling & Healing* and mention it here because children also dream of life after death and may need to have this aspect of their dream life acknowledged and respected.

Dream Sharing

Jacob's Dream

Jacob was running away from his brother Esau... Then when it was nearly dark, he came to a special holy place where his brother wouldn't follow him. He knew that he'd be safe there until the morning so he found himself a smooth stone to use as a pillow. He settled himself down and soon fell asleep. While he was sleeping he had a dream. In the dream he saw some stairs which led from his pillow right up into the sky. A glorious, bright light shone on this stairway and he saw lots of angels climbing up and down. He was amazed at the sight, then he dreamed that God was standing right next to him telling him that wherever Jacob went, God would be by his side and would take care of him.

- What do you think Jacob felt when he woke up?

- What do you think the angels were doing?

- Have you ever had a dream where a voice spoke to you?

Dream Sharing

More about Jacob's Ladder

Activities

- Draw the dream

Connections between earth and heaven.

- In Jacob's dream he had a ladder to connect earth and heaven. What else could be used to join them?

I thought of:

bridges,

rainbows,

plants such as the one in 'Jack and the Beanstalk',

rockets.

Angels

> 'When I was about five years old I was ill and I dreamt that an
> angel appeared in the room and my mother explained to her
> about my illness. She gave a blessing and I was instantly cured. In
> reality I was a little better the day after the dream.'
>
> Ashley (13)

Defined as spiritual beings who mediate between god and man, angels
have appeared in many dreams. Joseph had a dream in which the angel
Gabriel appeared and told him that Mary was pregnant and that she would
give birth to a son who was to be named Jesus.

> 'I dreamt I was Jesus' first angel.
> Jesus was welcoming me. I was so proud of myself.'
>
> Pattie (7)

In Martin Grimmitt *et al.'s* book *A Gift to the Child* a teacher relates her
experience of lessons on angels and dreams. When reflecting on the work
on dreams that she had done with her pupils, she said:

> There is such a bond between me and the children now, especially
> after the angels work when we shared our dreams. The children
> are more ready to talk about their beliefs, their inner selves, much
> more willing to share on a deeper level than before. Many parents
> have noticed it too, how the children have been so open, so frank
> about things. The benefits are intangible but so great and go on
> and on.

Milly (12), from Lancashire, dreams that she has a guardian angel who sits
at the end of the bed to protect her through the night; while the happiest
dream of Adrian (12) is of being in heaven with all his 'dead and live rela-
tions'. He described one of these dreams:

> 'We are floating. We float on a bubble of sugar. In the bubble we
> see a light of bluish colour... I see my face in it. I look happy.
> Then I wake up.'

These dreams give him a chance to re-experience pleasurable contact with
relatives who have died and are a source of solace.

Lucid dreaming

Lucid dreaming is different from ordinary dreaming in that the dreamer knows he is dreaming while still in the REM state. Out of this awareness comes the ability to control the dreams. He can direct the action, choose what happens in the dream and take off – often into flying dreams.

Celia Green, Director of the Institute of Psycho-Physical Research in Oxford, first coined the term 'lucid dreams', though it is not a new phenomenon. A 19th century nobleman, the Marquis de Saint-Denys, published the classic *Dreams and How to Guide Them*, which was all about dream control. Other cultures advocate the use of lucid dreaming: Tibetans practise a controlled dreaming for divination and healing, and in Malaya there are dream schools where Senoi children learn how to conquer their night-time fears.

The Senoi Indians of Malaysia practise and develop dream control as part of their culture. Their peaceful community owes much to the fact that from the earliest possible age children are encouraged to speak about their dreams and pay heed to them. If the child experiences fear in a dream he is asked to describe it, to speak of the fearsome animal or monster and to act out the dream. Members of his family and friends take on roles and ways are found which could help the young person deal with the frightening situation. He is then encouraged to confront the danger should it appear in his next dream. The basic principle is that if he confronts danger in his dream life he will overcome it in his waking life. This is a technique we can use with our own children.

The ability to control dreams often begins in childhood. Some children have a brief snatch of lucidity in disturbing dreams where, still in the dream, they say to themselves, 'It's only a dream, I can wake up', and they do wake themselves up.

Psychic phenomena and dreams

Psychic phenomena have intrigued and baffled humankind for centuries. In 2000 BC the Egyptian papyrus of Deral-Madineh gave examples of divine revelation in dreams, and oracular dreams were considered when decisions were made about matters of state. Most of the dreams that have been passed down from antiquity are prophetic, though a few are telepathic in nature. Frederick Myers, lecturer in classics at Cambridge University, introduced the word *telepathy* – from the Greek root *tele* meaning distant and *pathe* meaning feeling – in the 19th century. Noted dream researcher Robert van der Castle found about seventy references to dreams and visions in the Bible, while in ancient Vedic literature from the Orient, dreaming was regarded as an intermediate state between this world and the next. According to American dream researcher Dr Kelly Bulkeley many cultures believe that the 'soul' can roam in space and see this world and many others.

In 1882 the British Society for Psychical Research was set up, and dream telepathy became a subject of considered scientific investigation. In 1886 three of its founders published *Phantasms of the Living*, a classic study of the paranormal. It quotes 149 examples of dream telepathy which had been rigorously examined and verified by strict standards, and while not all these dreams would meet present standards of modern investigative criteria, a great many would. The characteristics of the telepathic dreams and their 'causes' are in keeping with what children told me about their 'strange' dreams.

Children may learn about psychic phenomena from television programmes, newspapers, books and general conversation but they also learn through personal experience. In my research into children's dreams I found many children spontaneously reported such dreams. Your own experiences will influence your reaction to this aspect of dreams, as will your openness to new data on the subject. However, as with all other dreams, listening to and respecting children's experiences in their dream life is as important in this area as it is in any other. Psychic phenomena in children's dreams are not rare. In a study undertaken by J. Prasad and I. Stevenson of 900 Indian school children, 52 per cent reported experiencing them in their dreams.

Many adults and children alike have said to me, when commenting on a dream that they regard as psychic, 'Please don't think I'm mad' or 'I'm really a sensible person, not weird or anything'. The taboo around psychic phenomena is still very strong.

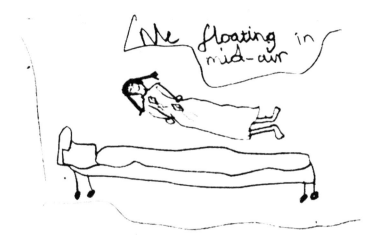

Floating in Mid-air

Astral projection and out-of-body experience

'Once when I was really ill, I started to float to the ceiling.'

Gary (10)

When I asked young people what information they would like to have included in this book, Poppy (14) said, 'I am totally fascinated by the astral plane and dreams about it. The prospect of the soul leaving your body during sleep is amazing. Maybe you could find out about a child's experience on the astral plane.'

An 'out-of-body' (OOB) experience is one in which a person feels he perceives the world from a location outside his physical body. Vivienne (13) told me about her first OOB experience in a dream. It carries a number of familiar hallmarks, such as rising above the body and looking down, and the shaking or jolting associated with the return to the physical body:

> 'I was in hospital and the doctors were operating on me and my spirit rose right out of my body and my spirit was looking right down on me. My body was dead but my spirit was alive trying to wake my body up and when my spirit returned to my body I felt the bed shake and woke up.'

Dreamers report difficulty sometimes in getting back into their physical body, or a disinclination to do so. Often they remark that a voice or person may tell them it is not yet time for them to leave their physical body. Such events begin in childhood but are often repressed or kept secret for fear of ridicule or disbelief.

Matthew (12) when he is ill dreams that he floats to the ceiling as if he is a ghost. The experience of being separated from one's body is recorded in the Bible, where in Ecclesiastes 12 a 'silver cord' attaches the astral body to the physical body, lest the spirit or soul become lost. Children report astral travel or OOB experiences while awake or under anaesthetic as well as during dreaming.

Dee, now 25, told me that since childhood she has had precognitive and OOB experiences in dreams. She remembered being chased, gasping for air, dreaming and yet knowing that she had to get back to her body. She was afraid to discuss this with anyone because she felt no one would listen to her. Nearly all of what she dreamt came true she said, which made her not want to dream; she thought there was something wrong with her. However, as she has got older she has learnt to accept and use her unusual insights. When we talk with children about their dreams we give permission for them to explore whatever worlds they dream about and accept the validity of their experiences.

> 'The car was on a bend when the crash happened. I don't remember us hitting anything, only the sensation being out of my body and soaring upwards and of knowing I was dead and wondering where to go. There was no pain and no panic.'
>
> Marisa (13)

Aileen Cooke, author of *Out of the Mouths of Babes*, reports numerous cases of children who have had both waking and sleeping psychic experiences. She tells of children, having travelled 'on the astral plane', each returning to their physical body with regret because, apart from not wanting to leave the beautiful world they discovered, they did not wish to take on the cumbersome burden that their body had now become. Others report flying through the air to see people and places, and being able next day to relate what was taking place far from their home, events about which they could not otherwise have known.

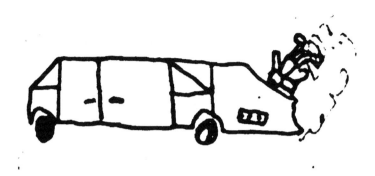

Boy Hit by Car

In 1962 a dream laboratory was set up at Maimonides Medical Centre in Brooklyn to investigate dreams and psychic phenomena. Since then hundreds of experiments have been carried out under the direction of psychoanalyst Dr Montague Ullman. What is fascinating about much of the research is that under rigorous scientific conditions, many experiments were significantly successful, particularly those involving dream telepathy, backing up evidence from other sources that extrasensory phenomena may occur during the dreaming state.

Anticipatory dreams

Precognitive dreams are those that concern an event that has not yet occurred. The dreamer may know that whatever it is will happen in the future, or may awake thinking that the dream was bizarre, odd or of special significance. Some precognitive dreamers comment that the quality of the precognitive dream, perhaps because of its vividness or a peculiar light quality, sets it aside from their ordinary dreams. Others have learnt that their dreams are precognitive or telepathic only after they have been recording dreams over time: looking back at diary entries they see the links between their dreams and waking events.

Anna (10) has many dreams about the future, mainly trivial events concerning her family. She talks to her father about her dreams as, she said ruefully, 'he is the only one that takes me seriously about my Forward-in-Time dreams'. As is often the case with psychic dreams, the content is to do with minor family concerns but the intense quality of the dream is quite different from her other dreams.

African-Americans, amongst others, have a strong belief in precognitive dreams. Traditionally, dreams have been seen as giving warnings and guidance. The great abolitionist leader and former slave Harriet Tubman dreamt of routes for the 'underground railway' (a network of safe houses) along which she took hundreds of slaves to freedom. When emancipation was proclaimed in 1863, she was completely calm, because, she said, she had already celebrated three years earlier when she dreamt 'My people are free! My people are free!', as Sarah Bradford relates in *Harriet Tubman: The Moses of her People*.

Gervaise (11), a partially sighted boy, had an unusual dream:

> 'I dreamt I got run over and the next day I did get run over. It was on a pelican crossing exactly the same as in the dream. I thought it was the dream again. I used to dream about hospital a lot after that.'

He may have dreamt this because of an unconscious fear of this crossing, or because of auditory clues (e.g. the sound of an ambulance siren in the background) that were causing alarm; or it may have been because of some kind of premonition. However, Gervaise, like so many children, does not speak to anyone of his dreams.

Many children who have dreams that later come true do not enjoy the experience. Rachel (9) put it very plainly:

> 'I have dreams that come true and I don't like it.'

Perhaps the fear is because some children believe that we dream so that the dreams can tell us what will happen in the future. They worry, usually silently, that the dream events will come to pass. Wendy (14) shows her anxiety about this:

'The most frightening dream for me is when I dream about something and the next day or maybe in a week it happens to me or somebody else in that dream.'

The best way to confront this anxiety is to assure children that though some people do have precognitive dreams, it is fairly unusual; and they can be very useful. Some people find such dreams helpful as they forewarn and forearm them; they act as an early-warning system.

One way to reassure the child is to ask him to keep a log of his dreams, which he can then check against waking reality. Armed with noted dreams linked to subsequent events he will be in a position to know when and if his dreams really are of the psychic variety. Encourage him to investigate honestly rather than dismiss what he says.

Hilary (11) told me that she dreamt of a flood in her home town of Strabane a few days before it happened. Fortunately Hilary was not harmed, but that was not so for Eryl. In 1966 Eyrl Mai Jones (10) insisted that her mother listen to her dream, even though her mother said she was too busy. Eventually she gave way and Eryl told her that she had dreamt that something black came down over her school and covered it. Initially she refused to go to school. However, in the end she did attend on that fateful day when, with 143 fellow pupils at her school in Aberfan, Wales, she was buried under black coal slag.

Eryl may have had an anxiety dream brought about by living in the shadow of the coal tip, but James Barker, a consultant psychiatrist, who undertook a thorough survey of premonitions about the disaster, judged it and many other dreams to be genuinely precognitive. In fact, Dr Barker was so impressed by the number of premonitions, involving people living outside Wales as well as in the local community, that he was instrumental in setting up the British Premonitions Bureau in 1967.

Delia, now 17, recalled her earliest precognitive dream:

'I was about 8 at the time and vividly remember a very disturbing dream in which my mother was screaming and there were several surgeons and lots of light in an operating theatre. I was watching but held away from her.'

When Delia was 9 her mother had to have a hysterectomy and was in hospital for a long period during which her daughter was not allowed to visit. Delia added: 'Since both my mother and I have precognitive dreams regularly it is discussed a lot in our home. It is not a taboo subject and is readily accepted by my parents and other relatives.'

Death

Dreams of the death of a member of our family may occur because subliminally we have recognised physical changes in that person. Where there has been no communication in the weeks prior to such a dream, it is much harder to explain how we can know of the death, especially when the time and details are so graphically incorporated in the dream.

Young children in particular may feel that if they dream of the death of someone, and it happens, they are responsible. When Rose, now an adult, was between 5 and 7 years old she used to dream about people before they died and saw their funerals. Many times her dreams proved to be correct and she firmly believed the deaths were her fault. Lucy (12) wrote:

> 'My grandfather was a very good sportsman. Two months before he died, I dreamt that my family and I were watching the regional news when there came a tribute to him on the TV. The tribute showed pictures of him playing football and other games, then at the end the presenter said "And that was a tribute to Robert Sidney W—,who died today at the age of 87".'

The dream gave her space to think about her grandfather and tell him how much she cared for him before he died. Lucy also dreams about hearing from a friend who lives far away and receives letters the next day. She commented that the quality of light in these dreams is different from that in her 'ordinary' dreams.

> 'When I dream about something it happens in real life a few days later. I dreamt my cousin fell off the swing in the park and he did. I dreamt about me and my friend going to Southport and the next day we went.'
>
> Michelle (11)

Of course, some of this can be explained easily: the child is looking forward to an event already known about. It is anticipation rather than precognition, but other dreams are not so easily explained. Elaina (15) spoke of two dreams which came tue. In one her mother had an accident and the sounds of police and ambulance sirens filled the dream. She was so disturbed by this that subsequently she would cry if she heard a siren while awake. Another time she had a nightmare:

> 'I was on holiday and eating in a restaurant when there was a loud bang and a man had jumped. Then I went on holiday in real life and it really happened.'

No one had comforted Elaina with the fact that such dreams have happened to other people throughout our recorded history, and in many cultures people who have such dreams are regarded as having special gifts to be developed, not hidden. If children such as Elaina can learn more about the nature of these dreams then she may well feel less at the mercy of them.

Telepathy

Many people believe that telepathy, the transmission of information from one person to another, mind to mind, over distance, without using traditionally recognised channels of communication, happens with adults and children. Jung saw telepathic dreams not as supernatural but as based on something inaccessible in our present state of knowledge. As we saw earlier, such dreams occur at times of great emotional upheaval, for instance at the time of death.

In his later years Freud became interested in the mystery of 'paranormal' communication, as biographer Ronald Clark points out. Freud conjectured that telepathy may be the original archaic method of communication used between individuals, and that as other sense organs have become more highly developed during our evolution, it has been pushed into the background. He put forward the view that such methods of communication could still manifest themselves under certain conditions. However, Wilhelm Stekel was perhaps the first psychoanalyst to observe that telepathic events have happened between people bound by strong emotional links, a view supported by research at the Maimonides centre in the USA. Telepathic dreams have also been recorded between patient and analyst, a relationship where the 'therapeutic alliance' or bond is all-important.

Retrocognition in dreams

Detailed historical-type dreams in children are defined by some as evidence of retrocognition, knowledge of time past, or a reincarnation from a previous life. Aileen Cooke in *Out of the Mouths of Babes* quotes the example of an 11-year-old girl who had a series of excruciating dreams in which she was held prisoner in the Tower of London and finally executed. The girl drew the axe from her dream – it was an unusual design – and asked to be taken to the Tower. There she saw an axe that was used for beheadings. It was the same design as the one she had drawn. Now, whether this is an example of 'cryptonesia', where the dreamer has come across such information when awake but subsequently has forgotten it, or whether it is an example of retrocognition or reincarnation, it is very hard to know. The author reports many more examples for those interested in following up this aspect of dream life.

We need to take the psychic and spiritual experiences of children seriously, and treat their remarks with great sensitivity. As Montague Ullman and Nan Zimmerman say in *Working with Dreams*, 'We are not only able to scan backward in time and tap in our remote memory, but we are also able to scan forward in time and across space to tap into information outside our experience.'

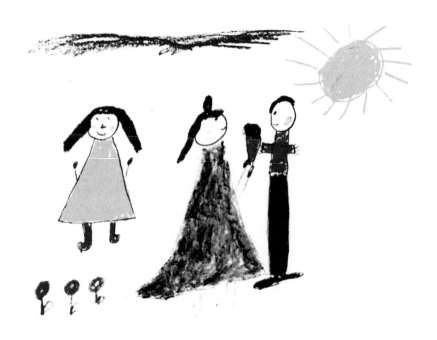

Ice Creams and Sunshine

Chapter Eleven

Dreamers' Delights
The Happiest Dreams Ever

A dream is a wish that our heart makes.

Louise (7)

Many dreams bring children enormous pleasure. Meeting fairies, eating wonderful food, flying around the world and being famous are the stuff of delightful dreams.

Now it is time to celebrate these dreamscapes with some of 'The Happiest Dream I Ever Had' as told to me over many years from children who have shared their dreams with me. In this chapter the dreams can speak for themselves.

Success:

> 'I am winning the dancing championships. I am an Irish dancer and I normally dream this just before an Irish dancing festival.'
>
> Shauna (11)

> 'I dreamt that I could fly and I went to visit Santa and the toys showed me the way to toyland I had a great time then on the way home, I dropped into Oz. They were casting 'The Wizard of Oz' and asked me to be Dorothy. I was about to meet the scarecrow when I woke up.'
>
> Emma (10)

'In my happiest dream I won an Olympic gold medal.'

Clodagh (10)

'I won the FA Cup for Liverpool.'

Ian (10)

Other worlds:

'I had a dream about sweets and everything was made out of sweets.'

Charlotte (10)

'I was in a coloured world and some rabbits asked me to stay for tea and I woke up laughing.'

Joanna (9)

'One day I was on my own, then I floated in the air. I could fly. I was flying everywhere.'

Zahoor (8)

'Tinkerbell the fairy, was outside my bedroom window with her friends.'

Andrew (5)

'I dreamt of fairyland…our beds were not made of iron, they were made of moss with rose petals for pillows and fern leaves for a cover. Just as I was going to sleep I awoke.'

Girl (8), reported in Kimmins, *Children's Dreams*

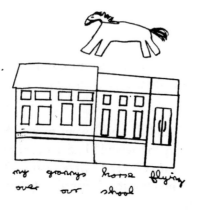

Granny's Horse is Flying

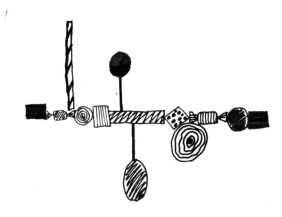

Sweets

Wish-fulfilment dreams:

> 'My happiest dream was one where I went to fairyland and they gave me three wishes. I wished that Conall was alive (that's a baby that I minded) and when I got back from fairyland I saw him rise from his coffin. But that was only a dream.'
>
> Eva (11)

> 'My happiest dream was when I got the bouncy castle to my house and I could jump from my bedroom window all day long.'
>
> George (10)

> 'On the night of my tenth birthday I dreamt that Mickey Mouse, who had turned into my uncle, threw a big party for me. He invited Alice and the Mad Hatter and everyone else.'
>
> Claire (10)

> 'The happiest dream I had was that I was with five stars dancing and singing. When I am grown up I wish that my dream would come true.'
>
> Janet (10)

Animal joy:

> 'The happiest dream I ever had was when I dreamt my hamster could talk and fly. She took me up to the clouds and we had a tea party.'
>
> Leah (11)

'I was in the desert with a kangaroo, I don't know why. I was hopping along because I'd taken the place of this kangaroo's baby. I was sitting in the desert with a kangaroo that had a hat on its head. It felt nice being the kangaroo's baby.'

Debbie (9)

Reconnection:

'My nan had come round to our house on Christmas morning and watched us open our presents like she always used to.'

Laura (12)

'I grow up to be pop star and have lots of beautiful horses and have lovely stables for them, and I have a lovely house for my mum and sister and dad – and that my dad came back to live with us.'

Jenni (9)

Relationships:

'My happiest dream was when I had a very bossy friend and she stopped being bossy.'

Annie (10)

'I was at school. I had a lovely coloured fish and I was a grand person and everyone was nice to me.'

Gemma (7)

And finally, a dream that saves the world:

'One day I dreamt that I woke up and we found that the sky had changed colour. After a week it still hadn't rained so we thought it was because the sky had changed colour. We decided to do something about it. We decided to get an aeroplane and go up with paint brushes and paint the sky back the way it was and then we'd come down, land the plane and we'd wait till the paint had dried and wait for rain. A week later it did rain. And as soon as it happened all the plants started growing again.'

Rebecca (11)

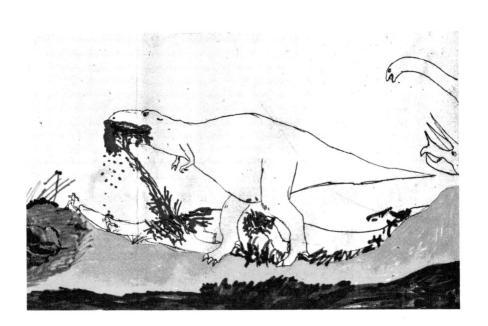

Dinosaur Attack

Sleep and Dreams
Books for Children

These books will help children to understand what dreams are and where they come from. They will help you to open up the topic of dreaming so that you can encourage children to share the joys and anxieties of their dream world.

The age divisions are merely guidelines; many books recommended for younger readers will also be suitable for much older children. You know your child best so be guided by that knowledge.

Age 5 and under:

Arnold, T. (1987) *No Jumping on the Bed.* London: Bodley Head.

Bell Corfield, R. (1988) *Somebody's Sleepy.* London: Bodley Head.

Brown, R. (1988) *Our Cat Flossie.* London: Anderson Press.

Collington, P. (1988) *The Angel and the Soldier Boy.* London: Magnet Books.

Gay, M.-L. (1987) *Moonbeam on a Cat's Ear.* London: Picture Lions.

Hague, K. (1987) *Out of the Nursery, Into the Night.* London: Methuen.

Hill, S. (1986) *One Night at a Time.* London: Picture Lions.

Howard, J. (1988) *When I'm Sleepy.* London: Andersen Press.

Hutchins, P. *Good-Night Owl!* London: Bodley Head.

Johnson, J. (1988) *My Bedtime Rhyme.* London: Andersen Press.

Kitmura, S. (1988) *When Sheep Cannot Sleep* London: Beaver Books.

Lloyd, E. (1982) *Nandy's Bedtime.* London: Bodley Head.

Omerod, J. (1982) *Moonlight.* London: Kestrel Books.

Age 5 to 9:

Carroll, L. (1989) *Alice's Adventures in Wonderland.* London: Puffin.

Dalron, A. (2000) *The Afterdark Princess.* London: Mammoth.

Foreman, M. (1982) *Land of Dreams.* London: Andersen Press.

Goode, D. (1988) *I Hear a Noise.* London: Andersen Press.

Impey, R. (1988) *The Flat Man.* Sherborne, Dorset: Ragged Bears.

Jones, A. (1984) *The Quilt.* London: Julia MacRae Books.

King, D. (2000) *Bear's Dream.* London: HarperCollins.

Lobby, T. (1990) *Jessica and the Wolf: A Story for Children Who Have Bad Dreams.* London: Magination Press.

Marshall, M. (1983) *Mike.* London: Bodley Head.

Mayer, M. (1983) *There's a Nightmare in My Cupboard.* London: Methuen.

Mayle, P. (1987) *Sweet Dreams and Monsters.* Basingstoke: Macmillan.

McCaughrean, G. (2000) *100 World Myths and Legends.* London: Orion.

McGough, R. (1992) *Pillow Talk.* London: Puffin Poetry.

Pavey, P. (1981) *One Dragon's Dream.* London: Puffin.

Pelgrom, E. (1988) *Little Sophie and Lanky Flop.* London: Jonathan Cape.

Pinkney, J. (1985) *The Patchwork Quilt.* London: Bodley Head.

Pinkney, J. (1987) *Half a Moon and One Whole Star.* London: Bodley Head.

Pomeranz, C. (1985) *All Asleep.* London: Julia MacRae Books.

Richardson, J. (1987) *Beware, Beware.* London: Hamish Hamilton.

Richardson, J. (1988) *The Dreambeast.* London: Andersen Press.

Riddell, C. (1988) *Mr Underbed.* London: Andersen Press.

Ross, T. (1988) *Naughty Nigel.* London: Puffin.

Rowling, J.K. (2000) *Harry Potter* Series. Bloomsbury.

Sendak, M. (1973) *In the Night Kitchen.* London: Puffin.

Sendak, M. (1975) *Where the Wild Things Are.* London: Bodley Head.

Seuss, Dr. (1962) *Sleep Book*. London: Collins.

Simmons, P. (1987) *Fred*. London: Jonathan Cape.

Wahl, J. (1988) *Humphrey's Bear*. London: Gollancz.

Wild, M. (1984) *There's a Sea in my Bedroom*. London: Hamish Hamilton.

Wilson, J. (1998) *Sleep-overs*. London: Doubleday.

Wilson, J. (1998) *The Suitcase Kind*. London: Corgi.

Wilson, Jacqueline (1999) *The Illustrated Mum*. London: Corgi.

Yabuuchi, Masayuki (1983) *Sleeping Animals*. London: Bodley Head.

Age 11 and over:

Blume, J. (1986) *Letters to Judy*. Basingstoke: Pan.

Dickinson, P. (1988) *Merlin Dreams*. London: Gollancz.

Duncan, L. (1983) *Stranger with My Face*. London: Hamish Hamilton.

Gleitzman, M. (2000) *Water Wings*. Basingstoke: Macmillan.

Lindsay, R. (1978) *Sleep and Dreams*. Donbury, CT: Franklin Watts.

Melling, O.R. (1986) *The Singing Stone*. London: Puffin.

Osborne, V. (1988) *Moondream*. London: Piper/Heinemann.

Pullman, P. (2000) *The Northern Lights Trilogy*. London: Scholastic Children's Books.

Shearer, A. (2000) *The Great Blue Yonder*. Basingstoke: Macmillan.

Storr, C. (1964) *Marianne Dreams*. London: Puffin.

Selected Bibliography

Ablon, S. L. and Mach, J. E. (1980) 'Children's Dreams Reconsidered', *The Psychoanalytic Study of the Child* Series, 35, 179–217.

Ames, L. B. (1964) 'Sleep and Dreams in Childhood.' In Ernest Harms (ed) *Problems of Sleep and Dreams in Children.* Oxford: Pergamon Press.

Ayalon, O. (1987) *Rescue: Community Orientated Preventive Education.* Haifa: Nord Publications.

Bass, E. and Thornton, L. (eds) (1983) *I Never Told Anyone: Writings by Women Survivors of Child Sex Abuse.* New York: Harper & Row.

Bettelheim, B. (1987) *A Good Enough Parent.* London: Thames & Hudson.

Bettelheim, B. (1978) *The Uses of Enchantment: The Meaning and Importance of Fairy Tales.* London: Peregrine.

Blume, J. (1986) *Letters to Judy: What Kids Wish They Could Tell You.* London: Pan.

Boa, F, (1988) *The Way of the Dream.* Boston and London: Shambala.

Bowlby, J. (1985) *Attachment and Loss.* London: Penguin Books.

Bradford, S. (1961) *Harriet Tubman: The Moses of Her People.* New York: Corinth Books.

Brody, H. (2000) *The Other Side of Eden: Hunter-gatherers, Farmers and the Shaping of the World.* London: Faber and Faber.

Brook, S. (1983) *The Oxford Book of Dreams.* Oxford: OUP.

Bulkeley, K. (1993) *The Wilderness of Dreams: Exploring the Religious Meanings in Dreams in Modern Western Culture.* New York: State University of New York Press.

Bulkeley, K. (1995) *Spiritual Dreaming: A Cross-Cultural and Historical Journey.* New York/Mahwah, NJ: Paulist Press.

Burton, L. (1974) *Care of the Child Facing Death.* London: RKP.

Chivian, E. (1983) *The Human Cost of Nuclear War*, Medical Campaign Against Nuclear Weapons. London: Titan Press.

Cohen, F. (1978) 'Art Therapy After Accidental Death of a Sibling' in C. E. Shaefer and H. L. Millman (eds) *Therapies for children*. New York: Josey Bass.

Cooke, A. (1968) *Out of the Mouths of Babes: ESP in Children*. London: James Clarke & Co.

Crick, F. and Mitchinson, G. (1984) 'The Function of Dream Sleep.' *Nature* 304.

Day, M. (1997) 'Britain's Forgotten Children.' *New Scientist*, 22 February.

de Becker, R. (1968) *The Understanding of Dreams*. London: George Allen & Unwin Ltd.

de la Mare, W. (1939) *Behold This Dreamer*. London: Faber & Faber.

Epel, N. (1993) *Writers Dreaming*. New York: Carol Southern Books.

Eron, L. D. and Huesmann, L.R. (eds) (1984) 'Television Violence and Aggressive Behaviour.' In B.Lahey and A. Kazdin (eds) *Advances in Clinical Child Psychology*. Vol. 7. NY: Plenum

Evans, C. (1983) *Landscapes of the Night*. London: Gollancz.

Feinberg, I. (1968) 'Eye Movement Activity During Sleep and Intellectual Function in Mental Retardation.' *Science* 159.

Fordham, M. (1944) *The Life of Childhood*. London: Kegan Paul.

Foulkes, D. (1977) 'Children's Dreams: Age changes and sex differences.' *Waking and Sleeping, 1*.

French, K. (ed) (1996) *Screen Violence*. London: Bloomsbury.

Freud, S. (1976) *The Interpretation of Dreams*. Harmondsworth: Penguin.

Garfield, P. (1984) *Your Child's Dreams*. New York: Ballantine Books.

Goodwin, J. (1982) 'Use of Drawings in Evaluating Children Who May Be Incest Victims.' *Children and Youth Services Review*, 4.

Green, C. (1982) *Lucid Dreams*. Institute of Psychophysical Research.

Green, G. *The Artists of Jerezin*. New York: Schocken Books.

Guilleminault, C. (ed) *Sleep and it's Disorders in Children*.

Greenberg, R. and Pearlman, C. (1972) *R.E.M. Sleep and the Analytic Process: A Psycho-physiologic Bridge*. Report to the American Psychoanalytic Association. New York.

Grimmitt, M., Grove, J., Hull, J. and Spencer, L. (1991) *A Gift to the Child: Religious Experience in the Primary School.* London: Simon & Schuster.

Hall, C. and Vernon, N. (1972) *The Individual and His Dreams.* New York: New American Library.

Handler, L. (1972) 'Amelioration of Nightmares in Children.' *Psychotherapy Theory, Research and Practice 9.*

Harms, E. (ed) (1964) *Problems of Sleep and Dreams in Children.* Oxford: Pergamon Press.

Hartmann, E. (1973) *The Functions of Sleep.* New Haven: Yale University Press.

Heather-Greener,G. Q., Comstock, D. And Joyce, R. (1996) 'An Investigation of the Manifest Dream Context Associated with Migraine Headaches: A Study of the Dreams that Precede Nocturnal Nightmares.' *Journal of Psychotherapy and Psychosomatics 65,* 216–221.

Huesmann, L. R. and Eron, L. D. 'Television Violence and Aggressive Behaviour.' In B. Lahey and A. Kazin, (eds) (1984) *Advances in Clinical Child Psychology 7,* New York: Plenum.

Jastrow J. (1888) 'The Dreams of The Blind.' *New Princeton Review 5.*

Jung, C.G. (1979) In H. Read, M. Fordham and G. Adler (eds) *The Collected Works of C. G.Jung* (1953–78). London: Routledge.

Keller, H. (1908) *The World I Live In.* London: Hodder and Stoughton/Century Books.

Kellerman, J. (1979) 'Behaviour Treatment of Night Terrors in a Child with Acute Leukemia.' *Journal of Nervous and Mental Disease 167,* 3, 182–188.

Kimmins, C.W. (1920) *Children's Dreams.* London: Longmans

King, N., Tonge B. J., Mullen, P., Myers, N., Meyne, D., Rollings, S., Ollendick, T.H. (2000) 'Sexually Abused Children and Post Traumatic Stress Disorder.' *Counselling Psychology Quarterly 13,* 365–375.

Kirtley, D. (1975) *The Psychology of Blindness.* Chicago: Nelson-Hall.

Kübler-Ross, E. (1983) *On Children and Death:* New York: Macmillan

Levitan, H. (1988) 'Dreams which Precede Asthma Attacks.' In Krakowski, A.J. and Kimball, C.P. (eds) *Psychosomatic Medicine: Theoretical, Clinical and Transcultural Aspects.* New York: Plenum.

Levy, D. (1945) 'Psychic Trauma of Operation in Children and a Note of Combat Neurosis.' *American Journal of the Disturbed Child 69,* 7–25.

Lewis, J.R. (1995) *The Dream Encyclopedia.* Washington DC: Visible Ink Press.

LoConto, D.G. (1998) 'Death and dreams: A sociological approach to grieving and identity.' *Omega: Journal of Death and Dying, 37,* 171–185.

Maisch, H. (1973) *Incest.* New York: Stein and Day.

Mallon, B. (1987) *Women Dreaming.* London: HarperCollins.

Mallon, B. (1989) *Children Dreaming.* Harmondsworth: Penguin.

Mallon, B. (1998) *Helping Children to Manage Loss: Strategies for Renewal and Growth.* London: Jessica Kingsley Publishers.

Mallon, B. (2000) *Dreams, Counselling & Healing.* Dublin: Gill and Macmillan.

Marner, T. (2000) *Letters to Children in Family Therapy.* London: Jessica Kingsley Publishers.

Martin, P. (1997) *The Sickening Mind.* London: HarperCollins

MacKie, R. and Whitehouse, T. (1998) 'This might be what be what God looks like: Moscow's boy in a million.', *The Observer,* 19 July.

Mellick, J. *The Natural Artistry of Dreams.* Berkeley, CA: Conari Press

Miller, A. (1991) *Breaking Down the Wall of Silence.* London: Virago Press.

Myers, F.W.H. (1903) *Human Personality and Its Survival of Bodily Death.* London: Longman's Green and Co.

Natterson, J.M. (ed) (1980) *The Dream in Clinical Practice.* New York: Jacob Aranson.

O'Neill, C.W. (1976) *Dreams, Culture, and the Individual.* San Francisco: Chandler & Sharp.

Petrillo, M. and Sanger, S. (1980) *Emotional Care of Hospitalized Children.* 2nd Edition. Philadelphia. J.B. Lippincott Co.

Postman, Neil, 'Violence: A Symptom and a Cause.' *Sunday Times,* 25 September 1988

Prasad, J. and Stevenson, I. (1968) 'A Survey of Spontaneous Psychical Experiences in School Children in Uttar Predesh, India.' *International Journal of Parapsychology 10.*

Proksch, K. and Schredl, M. (1999) 'Impact of Parental Divorce on Children's Dreams.' *Journal of Divorce and Remarriage 30,* 71–82.

Robinson, E. (1977) *The Original Vision.* Oxford: The Religious Experience Research Unit.

Rossi, E.L. (1972) *Dreams and the Growth of Personality: Expanding Awareness in Psychotherapy.* New York: Pergamon Press.

Sabini, M. (1981) 'Dreams as an Aid in Determining Diagnosis, Prognosis, and Attitude Towards Treatment.' *Psychotherapy and Psychosomatics 36.*

Saint-Denys, H. (1982) *Dreams and How to Guide Them.* London: Duckworth.

Saline, S. (1999) 'The Most Recent Dreams of Children Ages 8–11.' *Dreaming, Journal for the Association of the Study of Dreams 9*, 2/3, 173–181.

Shafton, A. (1999) 'African-Americans and Predictive Dreams.' *Dream Time Magazine.* The Association for the Study of Dreams 16.

Smith, R.C. (1984) 'A Possible Biologic Role of Dreaming.' *Psychotherapy and Psychosomatics 41*, 167–176.

Stekel, W. (1943) *The Interpretation of Dreams.* New York: Liveright.

Stevens, A. (1996) *Private Myths: Dreams and Dreaming.* Harmondsworth: Penguin.

Stevenson, R.L. (1983) In S. Brook (ed) *The Oxford Book of Dreams.* Oxford: OUP.

Tanner, A. (1979) *Bringing Home Animals.* New York: St Martin's Press

Terr, L. 'Nightmares in Children.' In C. Gillemault (ed) *Sleep and Its Disorders in Children.* New York: Raven Press

Treasure, J. (1997) *Anorexia Nervosa: A Survival Guide for Families, Friends and Sufferers.* Hove: Psychology Press.

Ullman, M. and Zimmerman, N. (1979) *Working with Dreams.* New York: Dell.

van der Castle, R. (1994) *Our Dreaming Mind.* New York: Ballantine Books.

Varma, V. P. (Ed) (1984) *Anxiety in Children.* London: Croom Helm.

von Franz, M. L. (1944) *C. G. Jung: His Myth in Our Time.* New York: Ballantine Books.

von Franz, M. L. (1986) *On Dreams and Death.* Boston, MA: Ballatine Books.

Wallerstein, J., Blakeslee, S. And Levis, J. (2001) *The Unexpected Legacy of Divorce: A 25 Year Landmark Study.* New York: Hyperion.

Wallerstein, J. and Kelly, J. B. (1980) *Surviving The Break-Up: How Children Cope with Divorce.* London: Grant-McIntyre

Weems, C. F., Berman, S. L., Silverman, W. K. And Saavedra, L. M. (2001) 'Cognitive Errors in Youth with Anxiety Disorders.' *Journal of Cognitive Therapy and Research 25.*

Winnicott, D. W. (1974) *Playing and Reality.* Harmondsworth: Penguin

Wiseman, A. S. (1986) *Nightmare Help: A Guide for Parents and Teachers.* Berkeley, CA: Ten Speed Press

Wolman, B. (1979) *Handbook of Dreams: Research, Theories and Applications.* New York: Van Norsrand Rheinhold.

Woodman, M. (1991) *Dreams: Language of the Soul.* Casette recording no A131, Boulder, Colorado, USA, Sounds True Recordings

Worden, J.W. (1983) *Grief Counselling and Grief Therapy.* London: Tavistock, Publications.

Yamamoto, K., Soliman, A., Parsons, J. And Davies, O.L. (1984) 'Voices in Unison: Stressful events in the lives of children from six countries.' *Journal of Child Psychology and Psychiatry 28*, 6, 127–33.

Yudkin, S. (1967) 'Children and Death.' *The Lancet,* 7 January.

Invitation

One of the joys of writing is hearing from readers. So please feel free to contact me with your comments and queries. Also, I'd love to hear about any unusual dreams.

If you would like details about training courses for individuals or groups, including school-based dream-work, please get in touch with me.

Brenda Mallon
7 Didsbury Park
Didsbury
Manchester M20 5LH
England
E-mail: lapwing@gn.apc.org

Index